Until We're Seen

T0265788

CONTEMPORARY ETHNOGRAPHY

Alma Gottlieb, *Series Editor*

A complete list of books in the series
is available from the publisher.

UNTIL WE'RE SEEN

Public College Students Expose the Hidden
Inequalities of the COVID-19 Pandemic

Edited by Joseph Entin
and Jeanne Theoharis

With Dominick Braswell

PENN

UNIVERSITY OF PENNSYLVANIA PRESS

PHILADELPHIA

Copyright © 2024 University of Pennsylvania Press

Published by
University of Pennsylvania Press
Philadelphia, Pennsylvania 19104-4112
www.pennpress.org

Printed in the United States of America on acid-free paper
10 9 8 7 6 5 4 3 2 1

Paperback ISBN: 978-1-5128-2637-1
Hardcover ISBN: 978-1-5128-2639-5
eBook ISBN: 978-1-5128-2638-8

A Cataloging-in-Publication record is
available from the Library of Congress

To our students,
past, present, and future,
and the insight and inspiration they bring to
our classrooms and to the world

CONTENTS

Introduction: When the Heroes Write Their Own Stories, What Do We See?

Joseph Entin and Jeanne Theoharis

The first months of the COVID-19 pandemic were filled with talk of heroes: the essential workers who kept our cities and country functioning. Daily applause and people beating on pots to celebrate front-line laborers rang out at 7:00 p.m., and hand-lettered thank-you signs flowered across New York City, the early epicenter of the pandemic in the United States. "New York State will go down in the history books as the place that beat back COVID," Governor Andrew Cuomo trumpeted on Labor Day 2020. "And when they write those history books, the heroes of the battle will be the hardworking families of New York."[1] But what if those heroes, those essential workers and their families, wrote the book themselves? What, then, would we see?

This is a book where the heroes tell their own stories. This collection features narratives by twenty college students—sixteen from Brooklyn College where we teach, and four from California State University, Los Angeles (CSULA), where our colleague Alejandra Marchevsky teaches—who wrote about their experiences and the experiences of their families and communities during the COVID-19 pandemic. These narratives are autoethnographies—a form of writing that marries first-person accounts with social analysis. These powerful, at times wrenching stories are told from inside communities that were hardest hit by the early pandemic's roiling health, economic, and social impacts, and then grounded in research to demonstrate their larger import and analyze their broader implications. They are not simply memoirs. The power of autoethnography is how these pieces, almost all of which were written during the white heat of the first two terrifying pandemic years of 2020 and 2021, become windows into complex social realities. They are keen examinations of how the processes of inequality were compounded during the pandemic and challenged by community mobilization.

The pieces included in this book portray a kaleidoscope of pandemic inequalities. Students recount cooking and handing out food for hungry neighbors, trying to aid an uncle who had been abducted by ICE and placed in a detention center that became a COVID incubator. They explain navigating the pandemic with a mentally ill mother, confronting their own mental health challenges that spiked during this frightening time, securing and distributing basic aid in immigrant communities, and delivering consumer packages for Amazon as the pandemic raged. They detail having both immigrant parents lose work due to illness and financial crisis, caring for an immigrant grandfather with worsening Alzheimer's, making handmade masks when an employer failed to provide any and then distributing them through the Puerto Rican diaspora. They describe helping a young child through online learning while taking classes online oneself, driving an ambulance through Brooklyn's eerily deserted streets, marching against police brutality, facing the fears of assault raised by the pervasiveness of anti-Asian racial hate. They document an entire extended family of "essential workers" getting COVID while simultaneously fearing deportation, helping neighbors in public housing by providing food and running errands, and watching an immigrant father die after catching COVID at his construction job. They are chronicles of harm, exploitation, and loss and also love letters to family and community facing some of the worst crises imaginable. They are the granular evidence of the devastating effects the pandemic has had on working-class communities of color, even as the United States has declared the pandemic over and looks away from its impacts.

This project began as a way to do something with and for our students that first pandemic summer of 2020. We teach at Brooklyn College of the City University of New York. When the spring 2020 semester was interrupted by COVID ripping through New York, it became clear to us how much our students and their families were suffering. Brooklyn College students are proud. Many of them come from immigrant communities for whom optimism is a lifeline to survival and success, and they do not always share what is happening to them. But the devastating health and economic realities leaked out. So many students and their families lost work, and the urgency for money was palpable. A student with a baby called, terrified to leave the house but having run out of food. Another student with multiple family members in the hospital texted updates as his father, too, was hospitalized. *Did we know of any jobs? Anything?*[2] The Brooklyn College food pantry was open but meager. *No halal food. Were there other options?* Students lost their housing; they couldn't afford food. *Could we help them access SNAP?* A grandfather was rushed to the hospital and then died. *He was like a father to me.* Family members were sick and coughing and coughing, students recounted, but they were too scared to go to the hospital, having no way to pay for it. *What should I do?*

Our impotence to help students that spring weighed on us. As scary as those beginning months were, we had protections our students largely did not have: salaries and health insurance, jobs that we could do from home, stable Wi-Fi, and rooms of our own to Zoom from. There had always been a gap between our social location and our students. But its wideness and what it meant for the safety of our lives and the vulnerability of theirs during the pandemic was palpable and terrifying.

Amid this deluge of fear, death, and economic pain, the Social Science Research Council (SSRC) announced a new grant initiative for research on inequality and the pandemic.[3] A rapid-response grant for scholars to begin to study the inequities that exploded during the pandemic, this needed to be research that didn't require Institutional Review Board (IRB) approval so that it could be completed and published in a timely fashion. We had an idea: to propose these students as the researchers to document inequalities playing out across the city. Hearing from marginalized communities themselves, from young people in these communities—and having those student researchers set the terms of the story rather than be included in short anecdotes or quotes—is exceedingly rare in general and certainly wasn't happening in the opening months of the pandemic. These young (and not-so-young) people are not the professional researchers that usually receive the funding to ask the questions and define the agenda. But these students had powerful stories of their own families and access to community experiences to document that didn't require IRB approval. They would provide a much different framing of the myriad ways that inequality was shaping and being shaped by COVID.

Part of the idea for our project came from having seen how research following Hurricane Katrina didn't include the communities most affected in the design of the research. Here again, we were worried about how inequality in the pandemic would be framed and studied. All too frequently, Black

New Orleanians became simply victims and objects of study and weren't included at the research table. Many researchers came in convinced they knew the questions that needed asking, often overlooking preexisting inequalities that had gone largely unaddressed by city and federal leaders. At times, they missed the organizing and the local, grass-roots institutions that anchored the community before and after the hurricane, largely casting Black New Orleans as people in need of saving. A similar tendency seemed present in much of the media coverage of the pandemic, where inequality was acknowledged but then the voices of people most severely affected were sprinkled as minor details while fundamental aspects of their experiences and community responses were ignored.

So, with Dominick Braswell, a recent Brooklyn College graduate (whose own piece is included in this book), we decided to submit a proposal for a pandemic autoethnography project for student researchers to analyze and contextualize what was happening to them and their communities.[4] To our delight, the SSRC funded our project. The grant enabled eighteen Brooklyn College students from deeply impacted communities across the city to spend the summer of 2020 crafting autoethnographies of their family and community experiences of the pandemic and receive $500. We held biweekly meetings on Zoom and a mini-conference so they could think through these issues together and bounce ideas off each other. Then-SSRC president Alondra Nelson attended our Zoom conference in the summer of 2020 to listen and talk to the students. As each student picked a facet of inequality to anchor their piece, braiding their own personal experiences with strands of research to amplify the context, the results offered a panoramic view of the various ways communities across New York City suffered, struggled, persevered, and resisted.

Powerful, poignant, and hard-hitting, their autoethnographies were deposited at the Brooklyn Historical Society, with SSRC, and in the Brooklyn College COVID-19 archive. But that didn't feel sufficient. The public needed to reckon with these perspectives. So what started as a small attempt to document the first months of the pandemic and put a bit of money in students' pockets became bigger. Eight of the pieces were shortened and published in the fall of 2020 in *Black Perspectives*, the award-winning blog of the African American Intellectual History Society. Out of this success came another cohort of twelve students in January of 2021 and a third cohort of nineteen in summer 2021.[5] Many of the students who participated were transfer students who had started their university careers at CUNY community colleges; we had met them in a Mellon-funded research program for Brooklyn College transfer students we codirect with our colleague, Alan Aja, who co-led the summer 2021 autoethnography group with us. Dominick Braswell helped facilitate all three cohorts with us. These three autoethnography projects were not classes; rather, they provided a chance for students to write, research, and share outside of the confines of a class with a stipend provided at the end.

Meanwhile, inspired by our project and confronting similar issues of students and communities at the breaking point, Alejandra Marchevsky, a professor at California State University, Los Angeles, decided to try an autoethnography project with her women's and gender studies students during the 2020–2021 school year. Marchevsky was Theoharis's longtime close friend; she had watched from afar the rolling crisis that hit New York City in the first months of the pandemic and how our students had used autoethnography as a powerful form of documentation and analysis. When things worsened in LA in the fall of 2020, making it the country's new epicenter, she saw the potential of this form for her own students. She decided to make it a class assignment.

In the midst of this, having seen the pieces in *Black Perspectives*, Alma Gottlieb, a series editor at the University of Pennsylvania Press, reached out. Had we considered a book of these narratives? No, we had not. Undergraduate research almost never gets published—and research by working-class students of color even less so. The Press was interested, inspired by the ways these autoethnographies reimagined the ethnographic project and the pandemic itself. The book would have to center these Brooklyn College student narratives, we insisted; it couldn't have elite faculty voices dominate or mediate their stories. And we wanted to include a section of CSULA narratives to demonstrate what was happening on both coasts. University of Pennsylvania Press editor Jenny Tan as well as Gottlieb understood the rationale and potential immediately. Thrilled, we began asking students; some were excited at the prospect of becoming published authors and having a national audience grapple with their stories and analyses. Thank you for this chance, they said over and over. Others demurred, not wanting their stories to be made public or not having the time necessary for revision.

This collective autoethnography seeks, at its root, to capture the impacts of the pandemic in New York City, the initial US epicenter, and Los Angeles, a later epicenter, on some of those cities' most hard-hit communities by community members. By reporting from opposite ends of the country for more than two years through diverse working-class public college student voices, this volume also captures key features of how the pandemic played out across the United States and beyond (some are transnational narratives that include people and events in Mexico, Pakistan, and Puerto Rico, too). The stories recounted in these chapters provide a detailed analysis of the hardships our students, their families, and their communities endured, as well as the creative, collective ways they supported each other to survive and keep going.

Working with our students profoundly shaped how we came to see the pandemic and its searing inequalities. These pieces tackle large social issues—poverty, precarity, racism, nativism, and the sacrifice zone, as Marchevsky explains in her chapter contextualizing the writings by her students at CSULA. But they do so by chronicling the small moments, the intimate or daily conversations and events in which the horrific forces of the pandemic struck—through the cruelty of a restaurant customer yelling at servers, through a corporation's callous disregard for the death of an employee, through the heartbreaking effort to reassure a young cousin that their parents would be okay when they might not be, through the attempt to memorialize in writing an undocumented immigrant family friend who was buried in anonymity. Equally important, students show the broader social realities these moments unveil.

Part of the power of these narratives, then, is the ways these writers get to choose not simply the issue to write about, but the terms of analysis. Autoethnography is not autobiography–it is writing that starts from personal experience, then identifies the research that will illuminate it, and lays out the analysis required to further understand a social reality. Part of the point of the project, we underscored with that first cohort of student writers, was to ensure a historical record—what future researchers needed to understand about the pandemic as seen, felt, and experienced by the students, their families, and their neighbors, coworkers, and communities. But these pieces were not merely raw historical data; rather, they were contextualizing and analyzing what they recounted, pointing future researchers not only to vital stories, but also to the questions that needed to be asked. A key part of autoethnography's power is the space it affords to investigate and unpack the broader social context of the writer's own experiences. By choosing the frame of their writing, these young scholars exerted a different measure of control and narrative design, expanding the bounds of what is included beyond an interview, interweaving issues that might seem separate (essential work and sexual harassment, gentrification and undocumented immigrant labor, public housing and mutual aid), and simultaneously erasing the scholarly distance from the issues described.

In response to the student pieces, four Brooklyn College faculty members—Alan Aja, Rhea Rahman, Donna-Lee Granville, and Lawrence Johnson—as well as Alejandra Marchevsky from CSULA, wrote short essays, framed through their own experience working with students before and during the pandemic. We chose these faculty because they are longtime advocates for students and for the mission of public education more broadly. From their various fields of expertise in anthropology, sociology, urban studies, political economy, gender studies, and Black and Latinx studies, they see students as people who bring with them a wealth of insight, perspective, and vision, *not* as people who come to college to get what they lack. These particular faculty are scholar-activists, deeply committed to student-centered pedagogy and to what students have to teach us as teachers, and our society more broadly, and whose own scholarship centers analyses of power, race, gender, and immigration. We positioned the faculty contributions as section responses and not introductions because we wanted to have the students, rather than faculty, set the terms on which readers encounter their pieces and the responses as reflections on the pieces and the research that each brings to bear.

The book's title, *Until We're Seen*, comes from a line in Samantha Saint Jour's chapter about her harrowing experience working at McDonald's as COVID-19 hit New York. Sammy suggests that until the pandemic is seen through the perspectives of the predominantly young, working people of color, we won't be able to adequately grasp or confront its layered, cascading impacts and what needs to be changed in our society. One of the themes that runs through the pieces is the ways that society tends to ignore these realities—to *not* see what is happening to people, especially to socially and economically vulnerable communities.

These pieces focus on New York City and Los Angeles because they became "sister cities" of the COVID-19 pandemic in the United States, the first two epicenters as the virus swept across the country.[6] NYC and LA share many characteristics that led to the virulence of the pandemic in both places: global economies with robust manufacturing and service sectors that require workers to be on-site with limited social distancing; extreme wealth inequality along lines of race, gender, nationality, and immigration status; large Black and brown communities that faced deep health vulnerabilities even before the pandemic; long-standing residential segregation and expensive housing markets that result in overcrowded housing conditions and homelessness; and underfunded and heavily used public infrastructure, including public health care, education, and transit, that have been depleted by decades of government austerity. It became clear as the epicenters of the pandemic moved across the country from New York and LA to pockets of the South and Southwest that COVID-19 was a story of how preexisting social conditions; the inequities of US racial capitalism exponentially increased a pattern of harm against already-vulnerable people and communities.

These accounts show that New York and LA were canaries in the coal mine, demonstrating that the pandemic *did* discriminate. While Americans across class and race contracted the virus, the patterns of harm, death, and increased economic vulnerability followed the race, class, and gender fissures endemic to US society.[7] By placing LA alongside the stories coming out of New York, this book demonstrates how these accounts are both particular and representative of what was happening to working-class communities of color across the country—from farm workers in the Southwest to meatpackers in the Midwest, from prisoners to home health care workers to delivery app workers. These autoethnographies show how capitalism's racialized patterns of exploitation shaped the ways the pandemic played out.

But the story of COVID-19 also demonstrates how communities stepped up, often in the face of state abandonment. This book offers not only first-person accounts of structural inequalities, but also stories of hope and persistence in which neighbors and communities—across cities and transnational diasporas—marshalled to try to prevent others from dying or going hungry. These stories of community mobilization, grounded in the recognition of our social interdependency, were absent from many mainstream treatments of the pandemic. They present a vision of what this society could be and how we could care for each other if we learned from the pandemic and what people built to protect each other.

Not the College Students You See on TV

The writers in this book are all college students or recent graduates of large, urban public universities. Brooklyn College is one of the twenty-five campuses that make up the City University of New York (CUNY) system, and the majority of our students hail from working-class and poor immigrant families and communities of color. Over half of CUNY students come from households that earn $30,000 or less, in one of the most expensive cities in the world. Eighty-five percent are persons of color; 35% are foreign born; 45% are the first in their families to attend college.[8] A study done *before* the pandemic found 48% of CUNY students experienced food insecurity within the month and 14% were homeless within the previous year.[9] Another study, which surveyed CUNY students in the first months of the pandemic, revealed that 81.1% of CUNY students reported loss of household income due to the pandemic and half (49.8%) worried about losing their housing.[10]

Like their CUNY counterparts, Cal State LA students are overwhelmingly (95%) Latinx, Asian American and Black, first-generation college students, immigrants, parents, and low-wage workers. In 2017, the median family income among Cal State LA undergrads was $40,300, far below HUD's benchmark for a low-income household in Los Angeles.[11] A study conducted in 2019 across the twenty-three-campus California State University system found students struggling to meet their basic needs before the pandemic: nearly 40% experienced food insecurity and 11% had experienced homelessness within the past twelve months.[12] This preexisting precarity was amplified for CSU students during the pandemic. In spring and fall of 2020, the California Student Aid Commission surveyed college students enrolled in a range of higher education institutions, from private to vocational, to track the pandemic's effects on their lives and education. Those attending a CSU were most likely to have a parent who was sick with COVID-19; about half of CSU respondents experienced a decrease in work hours and increase in monthly housing and food expenses and one-third reported changes to their housing situation due to the COVID-19 pandemic.[13]

It is not just our students who are poor and working class. Both Brooklyn College and CSULA are large, urban, working-class-serving universities that have been chronically starved of funding. CUNY, which is funded jointly by the city and state, has suffered decades of underfunding under both Democratic and Republican governors and mayors. CUNY was free to attend for its first 130 years. Tuition was implemented during the mid-1970s, just as CUNY was becoming a majority-BIPOC-serving institution, and now constitutes 40% of the university's budget. Similarly, at Cal State, the state's share of the operating budget has dropped from 80% in the mid-1990s to 60% today.[14] The impacts of long-standing, inadequate state funding are ubiquitous, from overcrowded classrooms with broken desks and chipped paint, to an overreliance

10   Joseph Entin and Jeanne Theoharis

on severely underpaid adjunct labor (adjuncts teach the majority of classes at CUNY), to leaking labs and inadequate study and social space for students. CUNY and CSU remind us that when it comes to education in the United States, students who have the least to begin with typically get the fewest resources. It's a structure of higher education that in key ways deepens rather than diminishes already existing disadvantages. Yet as the pieces in this volume attest, our students persevere in the face of underfunding, savoring the opportunities to study, think, and create that these public universities provide.

Written by CUNY and CSU students, this book provides a very different window into college pandemic life than we are used to seeing. Many of the portrayals of college under COVID picture the 2020 closing of dorms and exodus from campus, the sadness of missing friends, students on laptops Zooming in from all parts of the country, and then elaborate testing protocols, dorm room isolation, and bad grab-and-go food that characterized many colleges' return to campus. The college experience chronicled in this book is far from that. Indeed, while the dominant image of college in our society remains the elite residential school, the vast majority of college students in the United States—85%—actually attend commuter schools.[15]

Because Brooklyn College and CSULA are commuter institutions, our students' educational experiences—deeply interwoven with family and work—already diverged from popular images of college life. A full slate of classes, minimum wage work, family and elder care, long subway (or in LA, automobile or bus) commutes, crowded living conditions—these were the typical components of college life for our students before the pandemic. Rather than being sequestered on an isolated campus, or caught in a town-gown divide, CUNY and CSULA students attend college as part of their everyday, urban existence, continually connecting campus, community, and city. Over half of CUNY students work while in school, and half of those work twenty hours or more per week, even as New York State's tuition assistance program required that students take five courses per semester to maintain their financial aid.[16] And the pandemic only deepened that precarious balancing act. Yet there are few outlets where we can hear from these students in their own voices and few stories in the media feature public university students, even before COVID struck.

For our students, many of whom are the first in their family to go to college, school has long been a hard-won and cherished goal. Brooklyn College is 21% Asian, 23% Black, 23% Latinx, and 29% white (including many white immigrant students, particularly from Eastern Europe) so our classes are a rainbow—African Americans and West Indians; students from Pakistan, Haiti, Yemen, and Russia; Uzbeki immigrants and longtime white Brooklynites; Orthodox Jewish students, Catholic Nuyoricans, and Bengali Muslims; gay, trans, and straight—talking, listening, and learning across lines that seem unbridgeable in other parts of American society. The kinds of conversations we have in class, the caliber of questions and breadth of research that students pursue, and the ways they listen and imagine the best for one another model what US society could be. The range of student clubs on campus and the ways students are embedded in religious, political, and social organizations in their communities capture the kaleidoscope of New York City's diversity.

The commitment of Brooklyn College students to education is palpable. Over and over, they tell us how much our classes mean to them, how they share the readings with their parents and kids, friends and partners. Over and over, they face harrowing times in their lives—homelessness, the death of loved ones, unsafe living situations—and still they show up with their readings done. Over and over, they work thirty or forty or fifty hours outside of school and take care of families and do their homework on the subway or in the early morning or late evening. Over and over, when we run into them, even many years later, they say they still cherish the course pack of readings from class and how much it changed the ways they understand the world around them. When given the opportunity to write about the pandemic's effects on their community, they shone. Imbued with a responsibility to document a story of their community largely not being told, they produced work even beyond our wildest imagination.

Brooklyn College and California State University-Los Angeles rank at the top of schools in the United States providing social mobility for their students, and our university administrations and public officials trumpet this fact often. Getting to be part of this transformation is incredible—a student who had never met a lawyer personally is now a public defender in the city, another who worked overnight all through college to support their disabled mother is now finishing a PhD, an older student who put himself through college now works for a major newspaper. Many of our students go on to be teachers, counselors, public servants, and municipal workers who maintain the social and economic fabric of this immense city. But our students' economic mobility shields a much more sobering reality: how poor our students and their families are to begin with. And the ways that the public officials burnish their accomplishments and persistence hides the systematic underfunding of public higher education.[17]

One of the hardest things for us as we sheltered at home in that first year of the pandemic was the national celebration of Andrew Cuomo. Cuomo had been devastating for CUNY, cutting CUNY's funding relative to increasing enrollments and rising costs *every year* he was in office. And despite organized campaigns by students, faculty, and the faculty-staff union, the public had largely been indifferent, reelecting him twice. The only time in the past decade that the *New York Times* did a serious story on the underfunding of CUNY and the dilapidated classrooms, crumbling ceilings, and nonworking bathrooms was on the eve of Michelle Obama's 2016 commencement speech at City College. In the weeks before CUNY finally moved to online learning on March 19, 2020 (later than many other NYC universities did), the decaying physical plant seemed all the more sinister. There had never been reliable soap in the bathrooms, the ventilation had always been poor, ceiling tiles fell, and pipes leaked. Some classrooms didn't even have a window and many barely had enough seats for everyone.

And then the transition online brought new challenges. The overwhelming majority of our students live at home—and often home includes not only siblings and parents, but also grandparents, children, and other extended family. During the pandemic, students had to consider not only themselves, but also the thick web of relations they were woven into. That vulnerable family members could be exposed was an ever-present worry; sheltering in an overcrowded apartment meant that private space was often nonexistent and "social distancing" out of the question. *I don't know if I can turn my camera on because there are so many people in the room*, was a common refrain. Zooming in from bathrooms or while tending to young brothers and sisters, standing outside McDonald's to grab Wi-Fi to finish their papers, writing assignments on their phones—this was college during the pandemic for many of our students.

What they missed most, so many students told us, was the library—a quiet place of their own to study, meet friends, and be themselves. It became clear in ways that we had never fully appreciated how school was not merely a hoped-for pathway to economic mobility, but something they were doing for themselves, a place to nurture and develop their own talents and intellectual interests and become the persons they wanted to be, amid competing family and work responsibilities and pressure from parents about what they should do or be. So the pandemic took a deep personal toll. The economic catastrophe that befell most of our students as the pandemic continued was also devastatingly clear. *My parents don't have jobs that pay for them to work at home. . . . I don't have a job anymore. . . . I have to find another job, or we won't have income.*

Our students had always come with too much stoicism, too much willingness to take whatever bad things happened into themselves and persevere. And that only grew. The pandemic brought so much apologizing—for the noise in their rooms, for not being able to turn their camera on, for not submitting assignments on time because they had been evicted or had family members get sick. Within higher-education circles, the idea stuck that students were disconnecting from school (particularly if their Zoom cameras were off) but *if* they were committed, they would be able to rise above. That was impossible but the impact of that dangerous idea on students was significant. Shamed for struggling, many didn't admit it. In the first months of the pandemic, only a couple of students confessed to us they didn't have a laptop of their own or access to reliable Wi-Fi. But surveys of CUNY students revealed that *more than half* didn't. When Brooklyn College started making small connectivity grants available, so many students were eager and tried to apply, even though the website for the grant often didn't work.

The hand-wringing about disconnected students and widening learning gaps was not our experience. They showed up, wrote in the chat, told us over and over how much this learning meant to them. With our colleague Alan Aja, we run a program for transfer students to conduct intensive semester-long independent research projects. In the first online semester, we worried: how would students continue researching? What would a research conference look like online? Yet the work students produced that term was impressive, their research intricate. The conference entailed five hours on Zoom and they were still asking questions of each other at the end. Their supportiveness was visceral; when one student got admitted to law school, the chat erupted into congratulations; when another student got nervous, the chat filled with encouragement: "don't worry," "you know this," "you got this." Every semester of online teaching, we worried: how do you make community online? And students showed us. They started WhatsApp groups to connect with each other and used the chat to have far-ranging class discussions, making watching films in class the most fun it had ever been.

This is not to say that teaching online was easy or always fulfilling. At times, it was exhausting, the black Zoom squares demoralizing. Figuring out the right balance of supporting students and pushing them felt unbearably tricky.

Some of our students dropped out and many struggled mightily—not because they didn't have the fortitude, but because the economics and the balancing of new realities were impossible. And we struggled too, forced to teach in ways that frequently felt impersonal and clunky. We missed the human contact and interaction of the classroom and found teaching online often disorienting and at times disheartening.

As faculty, one of the hardest things in doing this work was realizing again and again how much students were keeping inside—students we'd had in class revealed more in their autoethnographies, and then more in conversation. There was so much we didn't know, and it became clear, so much they were carrying. Some students included details in initial drafts but took them out in the final version because they were too personal. Even with the rawness of the pieces gathered here, there is so much these young people did not include. But that is part of the point. The power here is in the details, the frame, and the reflection, which unveil more viscerally a particular social reality. This is not tragedy porn, not a prurient view from the outside, but analysis grounded in first-person experience. Most of the pieces show the conditions of inequality before the pandemic that widened and worsened. Ultimately, they demonstrate a social reality that could be different and the work we must all do to change it.

Inequality at the Epicenter

The initial context for our students' writing was the particular force with which the first wave of the pandemic hit New York City both in sickness and in economic devastation. During the early phase of the outbreak, in March and April 2020, NYC accounted for almost half of the total cases in the United States.[18] By May 2020—just two months into the pandemic—there had been almost thirty thousand deaths.[19] In the first nine months of the pandemic, Latinx and Black New Yorkers died from COVID-19 at twice the rate of white New Yorkers.[20] Just like the racial disparities in health outcomes, the economic fallout disproportionately hurt New Yorkers of color. Black New Yorkers were 51% more likely than white New Yorkers to report a job loss or reduced hours due to the pandemic. Latinx and Black New Yorkers were 1.3 to 2 times more likely than white New Yorkers to report financial difficulties such as paying for rent, gas, electricity, phone or internet bills, public transportation, and groceries.[21] Fifty-four percent of immigrants employed in the private sector lost jobs during the pandemic.[22]

Even among the employed, immigrant and BIPOC NYC residents were more likely to be front-line workers, which increased the risk of COVID-19 exposure, and were also less likely to have paid sick leave.[23] Fewer than half of undocumented immigrants in NYC reported that they were able to receive the medical care they needed due to factors such as the paucity of language services (translators), crowded local hospitals, and a lack of health insurance.[24]

COVID-related business closures and unemployment left people of color vulnerable in the area of housing as well. A 2020 study found that Asian, Black, and Latinx tenants in NYC were three to four times more likely than whites to be behind in rent payments.[25] As a 2021 study published in the *Journal of Urban Health* explained, these economic conditions led to further health inequity: people "at the highest risk of eviction are also more likely to live in substandard housing conditions that threaten their health, such as poor ventilation, pest infestations, and mold—all closely associated with the development of respiratory conditions and general poor health."[26] Low-income communities riddled with hunger and food insecurity also saw emergency food programs disappear as the city went into lockdown. Thirty-eight percent of soup kitchens and food pantries were closed by mid-April 2020.[27] Racial capitalism's jagged landscape of social and economic disparities ensured that COVID would play out in grotesquely uneven ways, compounding the preexisting vulnerabilities that marked working-class communities of color.

On top of this, the pandemic ushered in intensified patterns of racial hatred and violence against people of color, especially Asian Americans and Black Americans. The number of racially motivated hate crimes reported in 2020 jumped 32% from 2019. President Donald Trump repeatedly referred to COVID-19 as the "Chinese virus," and anti-Asian violence rocketed up 77% from 2019 levels, according to the US Justice Department; the following year was much worse, as hate crimes against Asian Americans soared by 342%.[28] In New York City, elderly Asian Americans were assaulted on the streets and pushed onto subway tracks. And a global pandemic did not arrest the drum beat of police violence against Black people; Ahmaud Arbery, Breonna Taylor, and George Floyd were among the 164 Black people killed by police in the first eight months of 2020.[29]

Even as COVID began to consume the rest of the country and New York was no longer the epicenter, the devastating impacts of the pandemic spiraled in the city over the next two years and beyond.[30] Many families kept working and even if they had managed to avoid getting the virus early on, months of work and exposure led many more New Yorkers (including many of the families in the book) to contract the virus, often multiple times. The collateral deaths and long-term health issues of the pandemic mounted. As temporary unemployment benefits expired and meager savings were exhausted, housing issues grew acute. To us as teachers, every COVID semester felt different, devastating in its own way, as students faced rolling challenges. Benefits ran out, new family members moved in, people were forced to move because their current housing became unaffordable in the face of economic losses, ongoing health problems left some family members unable to work. The stress and sadness were ever present, and the government response anemic: two rounds of federal checks and a year of eviction protection was not enough to protect poor and working-class people from the economic catastrophe of the pandemic's layered effects. At the same time, New York's (and the world's) rich grew richer—in some cases astronomically so.[31]

Almost two years after the initial wave, as CUNY prepared to return to classrooms in spring 2022 for the first time since March 2020, Omicron hit. CUNY barreled forward, alongside NYC's public schools, despite other colleges in the New York area postponing in-person classes to let the wave die down. New York City's new mayor, Eric Adams, urged people to stop "wallowing in COVID" and get "back to normal" in the face of sky-high rates of infection across the city.[32] This celebration of "resiliency," the insistence that "New York is back," implied that those who didn't make it simply weren't resilient enough—that it was about attitude, rather than an ever-widening economy and a still-spiraling health crisis exacerbated with many people uninsured. That fetish of individualism—that whatever happens to you or your family is now on you—only worsened as Biden declared the pandemic over and then ended it as a "national emergency" in May 2023. The city is now no longer tracking COVID rates, but wastewater testing confirmed that in the winter of 2024, the virus was still circulating widely.[33]

Documenting the Hardship and Also the Love

In recounting 2020, 2021, and 2022 through the experiences of predominantly young, working-class immigrants and people of color, these autoethnographies present a different story of pandemic New York City and Los Angeles, and the nation more broadly, than the dominant public understandings of the pandemic. All of the student writers in this book are Black, Latinx, and/or Asian American. The *New York Times* ran stories about offices shuttering, residents fleeing the city (and then later, articles wondering "will they return?"), subway use plummeting, as well as particularly egregious articles like "Turning Your Second Home into your Primary Residence."[34] That was not the experience of our students (even though they, too, are *New York Times* readers). Very few of these students and their families had the luxury of working from home; if they were able to keep their jobs, they took subways and buses and worked. They drove delivery trucks, worked in private homes, cooked food in restaurants for people to pick up, and worked at grocery and other retail stores. They couldn't leave; if anything, more people moved in, as family members unable to pay for housing were forced to consolidate to save money.

The economic, medical, and social catastrophe of the pandemic reverberated through students' lives; when family members lost jobs or took sick, it resounded through the whole household. The fear was ever-present, of COVID, of job loss, of not having health insurance. Some students took on new jobs to help their families; others lost jobs and struggled to find work; many others kept their "essential" jobs and worried constantly about exposure to COVID and whether they would bring the virus home to parents and grandparents (many immunocompromised). And when they did get COVID, or someone in their family got it (and most did), quarantining was next to impossible. And sick days—well, that was an upside-down idea: not only did many students and their families not get paid when they stayed home sick (even if they were allowed to) but they often didn't have access to health insurance either.

To be sure, these are stories of hardship and loss, of illness and sadness and despair. These pieces recount the unadorned predations of American capitalism and the gaping holes in the safety net of unemployment benefits, public assistance, and health insurance.[35] Yet these state failures were not simply unfortunate by-products of an unforeseen crisis. Rather, they were built on decades of chipping away at the US social safety net and converting the responsibility for systemic harm onto individual behavior. From Reagan's excoriation of "welfare queens" to Bill and Hillary Clinton's celebration of welfare reform's promise to move people from "dependency to dignity," the dismantling of the New Deal state had turned on blaming poor people and people of color for what befell them, and thus redoubling their vulnerability.[36] There was little net to catch people even before March 2020—and then the pandemic struck.

To some extent, the pandemic showed it was possible to protect and support people: the government could send stimulus checks and COVID tests, extend unemployment benefits, and halt evictions. But these efforts didn't lead to institutionalized, structural change or even the continuation of such benefits. New legislation ensuring sick days, hazard pay, living wages, and universal health care wasn't passed. Thus the stories of isolation told in this book are not about quarantining alone, but of isolation from government protection, as Alan Aja notes in his chapter. They recount what our CUNY colleague Ruth Wilson Gilmore calls the "organized abandonment" of working-class, poor, and immigrant communities, and communities of color by local, state, and federal institutions.

Meanwhile, the state continued to police, punish, and deport. The video of police officer Derek Chauvin kneeling on George Floyd's neck was both another example in a long and winding trail of police violence against Black people and also a palpable metaphor of the expendability of Black life in the first months of the pandemic where Black and Latinx people were working to protect, feed, and serve white lives, and dying at higher rates. In response, movements erupted through the city and the nation and also at CUNY, making connections between policing and living wages, between the need for Asian American studies and health care. An Anti-Racist Coalition was born at Brooklyn College of faculty, staff, and students, as Rhea Rahman details in her chapter, taking on issues from the decreased support for BC's historic Puerto Rican and Latino Studies Department to the need for Asian American Studies, to the over-policing of Black students on campus to Black staff promotion.

Yet if these are tales of hardship, they are also love stories—of students' families, biological and chosen—and of the deep resolve, mundane tasks, and herculean efforts such love entails. From Billie-Rae Johnson's decision to move back in with her mother to Genesis Orea's translating for her parents at the doctor's office to Anthony Vazquez's trip to Mexico to help his deported uncle, these are stories of family ties and cross-generational connections that made the pandemic very different from the "social distancing" and private "quarantining" that became dominant images in the first year. Together, these narratives testify to the importance of family and community and the lengths young people go to keep their families safe, secure, and functioning.

These stories are also testimonials to community power where mutual aid and organizing filled in when the state failed. They show what people were able to imagine and create to care for each other—and their pride in these community efforts. They are also a space to document difficult realities for young people who have grown up in families and cultures that say, "Don't talk about the hard things; focus on where you're going." And sometimes they are stories of fear or pain about the very families they were sheltering with and the gendered, homophobic, and heteronormative pressures that grew during the pandemic. The pieces in this book confront the hard facts of pandemic death, survival, and struggle, but on terms the writers choose. Echoing a phrase from Black organizing in New Orleans, they insist: *this is a history of what happened to us told by us.*

Beyond the Numbers: The Power of Autoethnography

Since the pandemic began, we have been inundated with numbers: in the United States as of July 2022, there were over 800 million documented COVID cases, and as of April 2023 more than 1.1 million deaths. Unemployment rocketed from 4% in March 2020 to over 13% in May 2020, and almost 15 million people lost employer-sponsored health care as a result.[37] But these numbers are dizzying abstractions, and it becomes hard to fully appreciate their impact and rippling effects. The narratives in this book insist on taking us beyond the numbers to focus on one person who died, one family without health insurance, one person deported, the toll of essential work on one young person. They unveil the politics of knowledge, of what (and who) gets recorded as important and what (and who) is made invisible, as Lawrence Johnson shows.

Look closely, these narratives demand. Sit for a while with us, these pieces insist. UNTIL we are seen, until WE are seen, until we are SEEN.

The stories collected here are the tip of the iceberg. As editors, we are achingly aware of the stories that did not make it into this book: the story of a daughter who spent hour after hour helping her immigrant father, a taxi driver, and his coworkers access unemployment insurance, but who could not also publicly share the tale of abuse she suffered at home; the story of a student who lived with six family members in a one-bedroom apartment, but whose chronicle of interpersonal conflict was finally too painful to put into print; the stories of mental health struggles that were too hard to write down in detail; the story of a Black mother navigating the pandemic with a two-year-old in a small apartment, and finding an outlet for her and her child in a local community garden, but who was in the end too busy to complete the narrative; the story of a powerful anti-eviction protest but then the friction and splintering of the group that occurred. For every hardship recounted here, and every moment of joy and collective resistance, there are others that remain unpublished and unwritten.

The stories that are included here are testaments to our students' commitment and endurance. They revised these pieces over months and years, not for college credit, sometimes after graduating and often on top of jobs and other responsibilities. Nonprofessional writers, they are mostly first-time authors who labored against incredible odds—in the face of poverty, illness, precarious labor, family obligations—to bring these narratives to fruition. These stories are powerfully crafted and made all the more remarkable because of the conditions under which they were written.

The temporality of these pieces is also intentional. They move between present and past tense to record experiences years earlier that continue to redound today. The pandemic and its effects are not over. While the pieces in this volume provide documentation for the historical record, this book is also not history. It cannot be relegated to the past. When we gathered the student writers in this book online in October 2022 to craft the conclusion of this book, they were clear: *this book is not a conclusion to the pandemic.* The pandemic was shaped by preexisting social conditions that must be grappled with if we are to understand what has occurred during COVID. In turn, the intensification of inequality during the pandemic will reverberate for decades, even lifetimes, to come—particularly if nothing is done to change it.

In addition to documenting the persistence, fortitude, and creative intelligence of individuals, families, and communities, these stories also testify to the power of autoethnography as a method and practice, and to the generative nature of collaborative thinking. Our project meetings—twice a month with the summer cohorts, twice a week with the January cohort—were important moments of human connection. Hearing each other's stories, talking about pandemic life in a group setting outside the parameters of grades, and reading each other's writing, allowed students to hone their own voices and also grasp the way their particular perspective added to a larger, collective portrait. It allowed them to push back on the messages about individualism and resiliency that heightened during the pandemic and to place their own family's experiences in a broader historical and structural frame.

Moreover, these extracurricular seminars gave students room to think and permission to experiment both with content and form (what mode of writing could best illuminate the issue they wanted to expose?). They had time to reflect, coming back to their pieces over and over, particularly as we worked to turn this project into the book. This sustained reflection meant that their pieces not only expose dynamics overlooked or occluded by most political officials and mainstream news outlets, but they also provide new lenses for seeing and thinking. They are scholarly interventions as well. Consider for instance Dominick Braswell's piece about life during COVID in one of NYC's public housing developments. Most scholarship on public housing tends to assume that "the projects" are broken and that residents want out. Dominick's piece asks us to reorient our vision: his piece doesn't shy away from problems—a result largely of decades of governmental neglect and underfunding—but his story's starting point is that residents build communities, that most do *not* want to leave, *that public housing is home.* Or take Daniel Vázquez Sanabria's piece on the pandemic's impact on his sister in Puerto Rico and the mask business she started to keep her friends, coworkers, and then others safe. Layer upon layer, the piece offers a meditation not only on family and mutual aid across the Puerto Rican diaspora, but also on colonialism, the Jones Act (and the ways it made personal protective equipment even harder to get on the island), and the solidarities forged between the colonial realities of Puerto Rico and the Navajo Nation. Starting with the story of one airport worker, the piece also asks us to see the pandemic in the expansive context of US empire and the networks of resistance forged across imperial borders.

Autoethnography, then, invites experimentation, which is reflected in the range of styles and conventions the contributors to this book take up. These stories are told as diaries, and as poems; they weave together intimate details and harsh realities with tales of hope and aspiration; they include small vignettes and litanies of facts and statistics. Writing against the grain, these narratives also raise difficult, challenging questions about what is seen, researched, and imagined, as Donna Granville notes in her chapter. What would it mean not simply to read but to use their ideas as the basis for policy? CUNY and CSULA students are not often viewed as part of our society's "thinking classes," but these pieces demonstrate the politics behind that. If students and their communities are viewed as deficient, then they are seen as the problem, rather than society. These pieces suggest collectively that our society is structured to render some people less important, disposable. What if these people and their families and neighbors had what they needed to thrive and were truly recognized for their "essential" contributions during the pandemic? As Lawrence Johnson asks in his chapter, what if our working-class, poor, and immigrant students were treated as knowledge producers rather than just knowledge consumers? What if their ideas and framings guided our collective path and policies forward?

Part of why we rarely see these kinds of narratives in the public sphere is because they implicate the American public in an uncomfortable way. They demand something, unveiling the self-serving comfort of the "Thank you, essential workers" signs that sprang up across the city. Faced with a crisis exponentially greater than 9/11, these pieces show in harrowing detail the ways our society continues to fail. As we finished the introduction to this book in summer 2023, President Biden has declared the pandemic over, but everyone is still tested before you get in a room with the president. Masks are off (unless you *choose* to wear one), the limited COVID benefits and Medicaid extension over, rent protections gone, mitigations in schools finished. New York City ended its COVID alert system just as cases were *spiking* during a new surge in July 2022. As these pieces attest, the new normal—unless we *do* something about it—is, if anything, worse, more callous, crueler and more unequal.[38]

These pieces ask us to bear witness to the violence of the normal which puts many people out of sight—from Billie-Rae Johnson's mentally ill mother to the undocumented worker buried on Hart Island whose story is chronicled in Yamilka Portorreal's piece to Maria Cerezo's construction-working father. There are so many forms of cruelty in this book—cruelty enforced by the enduring structures of racial capitalism and supported by the indifference and refusal to witness by so many Americans. Witness refuses the distance of merely seeing; we are implicated in what we witness.

Bearing witness acknowledges and acts on the interdependencies that link us to one another. *You are, therefore, I am.* These pieces express anger—and ideally elicit anger as well. CUNY and CSULA students understand the way society's arrangements are stacked against them; writing and research helped them find the hard facts and the *mots justes* to make those discriminatory dynamics concrete. To reckon with what these pieces bring forth is to absorb that outrage for ourselves, grasp the ways we are implicated in the problems elucidated here, and begin to work to fashion a different society. We hope these students' pieces can serve as a guide for that collective work for change.

We have organized the autoethnographies in this book into five categories: Essential Work, Disposable Workers; Race and Family; Crises of Health and Housing; Community Organizing, Mutual Aid and Struggle; and Gender, Sexuality, and Inequality in Los Angeles. This arrangement, however, is a bit arbitrary since most pieces could fit in multiple sections. Each section is followed by a reflection from a faculty member (the first four contain the Brooklyn College student narratives and reflections from BC faculty while the fifth contains the narratives from LA with a reflection from CSULA professor Marchevsky). We wanted these to come after the student pieces to model the format of a conference respondent, rather than suggest how to read the chapters.

None of these chapters are single-issue pieces. A story about labor and losing jobs is also a story about families, and about health and crowded living conditions, and about helping each other out. Audre Lorde noted that "There is no such thing as a single-issue struggle because we do not live single-issue lives."[39] These pieces confirm this insight. They also speak to each other in powerful ways, affirming and complicating and expanding each other's stories.

We hope that as you read, the effect will be cumulative, that each story will stand out for its distinct voice and images and research, and yet together they will change the way you think about the impact of the pandemic in the United States and about the way our society is structured. They raise the questions and highlight the many facets we need to understand to make the kind of transformational change that these pieces insist is so urgently needed.

PART I

Essential Work,
Disposable Workers

CHAPTER 1

Until We're Seen

Samantha Saint Jour

Waking up abruptly at 6:13 a.m., I get dressed in my McDonald's manager's uniform. I rush to work, fortunately just a few blocks away. I apologize to my boss for being late, wash my hands, take my temperature, write it down, and clock in. Once I leave the office to get ready to work, a woman comes in. She does not have a mask on.

"I'm sorry ma'am, I cannot take your order unless you have a mask," the cashier declares.

"Why do I have to wear a mask? I'm getting one drink, take my order now," she replies.

Realizing I have to step in, I respond, "Miss, our policy is no mask, no order. This has been decided by the owner of the store as well as the governor of New York. We have masks and can give you one if you do not have one."

The woman proceeds to curse me out, bang on the counter, and ridicule me, telling me I'll never amount to anything; it's nothing I hadn't heard before. I worked in fast food after all.

If you're wondering if she got her drink, she didn't. She couldn't get under my skin enough to make me give in, but she definitely reminded me that even though minimum-wage workers are "essential workers," working through the pandemic to provide food and supplies, we will never be treated as essential. Our importance is constantly overlooked, even when we're the last ones around providing necessities. Those working in the fast-food industry and in other minimum-wage jobs are accustomed to such harsh and harassing treatment since we work in a sector that does not even require a high school diploma. One would think we would receive the same celebration as everyone else who continued working through the pandemic, but society does not appreciate actual workers and their sacrifices; what is celebrated is the *idea* that there are people doing jobs that most people don't want to do—essential work.

For the five months I worked at McDonald's during the pandemic, I was scared of catching COVID-19 and spreading it to my family. When my father got COVID-19, I was terrified that I was the reason. I was the one continuing to work, coming in contact with random customers who barely wore masks. Every day, a coworker would catch the virus, and I couldn't stop myself from thinking about the times I worked with them, if I would work with them again, and if I had caught it, too. My coworkers who didn't catch COVID would come to me, asking why their hours were being cut. I had to explain to them that we could only have six to eight people working each shift to follow social distancing policies. They told me we were all better off receiving unemployment benefits because it paid more per week than our job did.

Most of the people I know work minimum wage. We all realize that just because we're considered "essential workers," that is not reflected in our pay, benefits, or working conditions. COVID-19 drew attention to the circumstances of low-wage workers, who are often young adults, women of all races, and people of color. According to the Kaiser Family Foundation, nationwide, 35% of minimum-wage workers are young adults (ages nineteen to twenty-five), 58% women, 23% Hispanic, and 16% non-Hispanic Black. These same groups average $11.80 per hour in pay.[1] Eighty percent of minimum-wage workers are paid hourly, which means if their hours are cut, their pay drops. While all minimum-wage workers get low pay, fast-food workers like me get paid even less—an average of $8.69 an hour—since it's not difficult to find people to fill those positions. The skills are easily taught, and no degree or education is required. Since I live in New York City, I was fortunate enough to make $15 an hour. It wasn't always this way—the struggle for that wage started in 2012 when the "Fight for $15" campaign staged its first strike in New York City.[2] Hundreds of fast-food workers walked off the job and went to the streets to demand a livable wage, improved working conditions, and the freedom to establish a union without fear of retaliation from their employers. It wasn't until December 31, 2018, when the minimum finally reached $15 per hour for New Yorkers. While this was a huge step, especially compared to what workers in other states were and still are earning, fast food labor has never effectively unionized. Unionization would allow workers to receive the benefits we deserve. In the remainder of the country, minimum-wage employees struggle to reach the level of $15 per hour due to regulations prohibiting the state from altering their minimum wage or political opposition to changing the minimum wage. It all boils down to a lack of urgency and concern for minimum-wage employees who are left to defend themselves.

Despite all the attention on essential workers and the data that was revealed because of the pandemic, no solutions were presented, just hollow words of appreciation from American leaders. The first step would have been to enact a federal minimum wage of $15 per hour, which is still not a livable wage. The second pandemic relief package under President Biden would have been a great opportunity to raise the minimum wage to $15, but political opposition in the Senate kept it out. The Living Wage Calculator reports that an adult in NYC with no children needs a wage of at least $20.42 an hour to afford their necessary expenses.[3] This demonstrates that the groups—young people, women, and people of color—most affected by the horrors that occur in fast-food jobs are underpaid even at $15 an hour. These are the same groups being disproportionately affected by the pandemic in other ways, such as mental illness, domestic violence, unemployment, and police brutality.

Many low-wage workers experience greater financial insecurity because of reduced hours, like my coworkers, as well as a lack of access to paid sick leave before and during the pandemic. To see if my peers were experiencing these insecurities, I conducted a survey of twenty-one random New York City students working minimum-wage jobs in different fields, such as retail, food service, and warehouse work. All respondents were college students of color. They provide a unique perspective on minimum-wage work and the intersectional issues that come along with it, such as racism and sexism. To reach the respondents, I sent the survey link to Brooklyn College club chats and posted the link on my personal social media platforms. I hit some roadblocks, such as inadequate response options, and some replies to the short-answer questions were repetitive or didn't answer the question. But the data I collected is illuminating.

Here are some of my key findings: 83.3% of respondents reported no access to hazard pay, sick leave/pay, bonus check, or any benefits while working during the pandemic. This is compared to a Pew Research Center study that found only 51% of workers earning $13.80 and 31% of those who earn $10.80 per hour have less paid sick leave.[4] Before COVID, at my job, if an employee was sick and did not find someone to cover their shift, they had to take a Tylenol and come in. During COVID, however, if you weren't feeling well, you were encouraged not to come in, and equally encouraged not to come back if you did not have a doctor's note. But you were not paid for missed time. Only corporate-run McDonald's, which are fewer than 10% of McDonald's franchises, had to offer two weeks of paid sick leave to staff who tested positive for COVID-19 in compliance with the most current policy adjustments introduced by McDonald's.[5] This goes to show that before and during COVID, minimum-wage workers do not receive any support for one of the most human acts—being sick. Along with this, 50.2% of respondents reported not having access to health care, and only 5.6% claimed they had health care from their job. If an employee becomes ill but lacks the means to recover fast, they miss even more work and are not compensated for it. It's a vicious loop that constantly sets minimum-wage employees up for failure simply because they're sick.

Finally, my survey revealed that 61.1% of respondents interacted with customers without a mask, and 61.1% also reported coworkers with COVID, demonstrating how surrounded minimum-wage workers are by the virus. They're always at risk of exposure, but when they do get exposed, companies do nothing for them, which is the equivalent of punishing them for something beyond their control, but well within the company's control if the right policies were in place.

Additionally, 1/7 of African Americans who are low-wage workers, and an even higher number of immigrants, fear speaking out against unsafe, exploitative working conditions.[6] I too was hesitant to speak out against another manager who was sexually harassing my coworkers and myself. Additionally, a new National Employment Law Project survey showed that Black employees are more than twice as likely as white workers to have seen potential workplace backlash against themselves or another employee for speaking out about pandemic-related issues such as lack of access to health care, sick pay, or unsanitary practices.[7] This stems from the absence of policy makers at all levels of government to do more to protect the interests of workers who are complaining about safety issues or refusing to work in dangerous conditions.[8] I didn't want to have my hours cut or get fired, and neither did the rest of the women I worked with. We're replaceable and we are reminded of that every single day by our boss, our customers, and the constant influx of new hires and decrease in long-term employees. But with effort, such as the one displayed in the "Fight for 15" strike, and the interest of policy makers who want to ensure that their constituents are safe, heard, and living a decent quality of life, essential workers could finally have the ability to lift up our voices, power, and bargaining rights.

Enforcing masks and social distancing policies were the most trouble-some experiences I had as a minimum-wage worker during the pandemic. It was hard for anyone to take me seriously in the first place; I was eighteen years old at the time, and a black woman, whether I was a manager or not. At my McDonald's, we put up signs saying "Masks required" at the door, the window, the cashier booths, and the pick-up stations. There were people who noticed the signs and would go back to their car to get a mask, but there were way too many who ignored the signs and came in anyway. My cashiers were scared to refuse to serve people, so they would take their order anyway and apologize to me for it later.

I understood why they were scared. At our location, a man attempted to throw a "Caution: Wet" sign at our workers and broke our TV menu instead. At our Coney Island location, a person pushed and broke our glass display. On social media, we saw employees getting punched in the face, spit on, and jumped for telling people to get a mask. People were smashing store windows and store property all because they did not want to wear a mask.[9] That could happen to any one of us, and I knew I could not protect myself or my coworkers. We all were on edge wondering when it would be one of us who would be assaulted for telling someone they needed a mask to be served.

About a month into the pandemic, my father was diagnosed with the virus. He works jobs he can't do from home: school bus driving and as a self-employed accountant at a firm in Flatbush, Brooklyn. He was working 6 a.m. to 6 p.m. on weekdays, until he caught the virus. I can't even remember if I noticed any symptoms before he was diagnosed; I was so caught up in working at least eight to nine hours five days a week, taking five classes, and keeping up with my mental health. I was so tired and sad all the time, I didn't even think of what was going on with the rest of my family.

Once my sister told me my father contracted COVID, everything fell apart. I was beating myself up for being so selfish, not looking after my parents, and for probably being the person who gave him the virus. Was I not sanitizing and washing my hands enough? Did I leave my mask or work clothes somewhere? How could I be so irresponsible? My father is the sole provider for my family, and without him I wouldn't even know what to do. Other minimum-wage workers I surveyed expressed the same worry of bringing the virus back to our homes where our elderly and young lived, or contracting it ourselves. If my dad had it, did I have it? My sister, as the oldest sibling, stepped up and took the lead. She told me to get a doctor's note, proving that I needed to quarantine for two weeks for everyone's safety. My job seemed understanding at first, allowing me to call out last minute and sending me a paid-time-off form. I filled out the form and sent it back; it was so simple. However, soon after, my boss sent out my shifts for others to take, which meant it would not show up as my hours, meaning I wouldn't get paid for whatever shift he gave away. I felt cheated. They were taking away the money I would have been earning, and needed now more than ever! These actions completely revealed a loophole in the sick-pay policy; if they changed the shifts I was scheduled for, then they were no longer mine and I would not be paid. Therefore, even with the right policies in place, companies can always find a way to just not give you the money you are supposed to earn, even during a life-changing pandemic. Between being worried about my sick father and my depressed mother, I didn't even have enough fight in me to demand my money back no matter how desperately I needed it. I knew my boss would say it was a business situation, nothing personal. Everything as an essential worker, however, is personal, since you are risking yourself and your family to make a living and survive. You're risking yourself so the corporation you work for can keep making money and remind you that you are expendable. When I clocked out and went home, I fell into a serious depression because I felt like I had no support and just wasn't making enough money to do anything. I was struggling to find a reason to live if it was just going to be like this—miserable even though I am trying to do everything right.

When I returned from quarantine, I heard many of the girls I worked with discussing a manager at our store. The manager, about forty years old and male, was taking their phones, requesting access to them to take a survey for the store (yes, we fake our surveys), but instead going through their messages and getting jealous if they were talking to boys. This same manager, before COVID, would put his hand around my waist, show up on my street, whisper in my ear, and randomly text and call me. Since I was gone due to quarantine and expressed to him that I was uncomfortable with his advances, he backed off, but it is clear he moved on to the other women, and had even more power to exercise such control over the employees because of the pandemic and the ability to blackmail female workers. I instructed them to go to our general manager; if they went as a group, it would be even better, but they were scared. They felt nothing would change and they might become targets of retaliation. Once again, I understood how they felt. Female minimum-wage workers (especially those in food service) across the nation are being sexually harassed despite all the harassment training. During the pandemic, this sexual harassment has become worse since employers know that employees need their job more than ever. Any sign of pushback was a one-way ticket to unemployment. The worst part is that not many report such harassment, especially women and immigrants, whether they are documented or not.[10] These groups will be vilified if they talk. With the job market so tight during the pandemic, low-wage workers feel lucky to be employed at all, and to complain is to risk everything they have.

There is no happy ending to this story. I left McDonald's, but my coworkers are still working for low wages, getting their hours cut, living paycheck to paycheck, exposing themselves to customers who might have COVID, getting cursed out by those customers, and withholding their concerns about the job. In fact, millions of minimum-wage employees working during the pandemic are experiencing all these afflictions as we speak. They are the ones waking up at 5 a.m. or going after their classes, and greeting customers who don't care about them or what they do. Minimum-wage workers are being kept invisible or silenced at work through blackmail or retaliation, and their concerns are rarely covered in the news media. This benefits corporations—even though they can easily replace workers, they can trap experienced workers into staying with the company for the same wage under the same conditions. This also benefits politicians, especially those opposed to raising the federal minimum wage, which has been stuck at $7.25 per hour since 2009. Raising the federal minimum wage and bringing awareness to the struggles of minimum-wage workers would eventually lead to the redistribution of wealth that politicians and upper-/middle-class citizens are not ready for. While there may be some discussion of the difficulties confronting minimum-wage employees during the pandemic, the only one highlighted is financial hardship, which may be the most critical but is not the only one. Our struggles are more than just financial; they are also about mental health, racism, misogyny, and classism. Minimum-wage workers are treated like second-class citizens who can be stepped all over. These are the same groups—people of color, women, and the working class—that have been oppressed throughout history; it is just a different method today. Policy makers and news outlets need to address the rapid multiplication of problems for minimum-wage workers instead of making it seem like money is the only issue.

Until we're seen as people who deserve to survive and have a decent quality of life, and as people who should be protected and accommodated for like white male workers in other fields, we'll have to accept the system that plays against us and doesn't give a shit about us, for $15 per hour or less.

CHAPTER 2

═════

Prole-ific

Zayd Brewer

I had always prided myself on being reliable. There's a notoriously low barrier for entry into the world of general labor, but even given that, I never felt comfortable doing the bare minimum. I was a delivery driver for Amazon, and the most critical part of that job was showing up, literally. The company I worked for, Touchdown Logistics, contracted daily routes from Amazon in the mornings and would then dispatch its fleet of midsize white cargo vans across Long Island and the outer boroughs of New York City to deliver whatever discrete necessities consumers desired. A common subject of the boss's ire was the frequency with which people would call out on days they were supposed to work. In the logistics business, the profit is in maintaining the fluidity of the operation and last-minute call outs meant Touchdown would have to forfeit the approximately $1,000 they made per route per day. The boss would threaten to cut days, fire people, cut hours, basically whatever he could, but people kept calling out and the impotence of his threats became increasingly pronounced. Guys took the job for what it was, a joke, and understood that the number of responsible people willing to endure the ritual subjugation that delivering for Amazon entailed was limited, an understanding clearly shared by the boss. When you're working as a subcontracted delivery person for the largest retailer in the world, even doing the bare minimum was unlikely to have many negative repercussions; but still, I had my pride.

This prideful adherence to an absurd capitalist paradigm did not strike me as inherently counterintuitive. In fact, all things considered I was satisfied with my work. Sure, some days were tough but generally my shifts were spent listening to whatever music I wanted as loud as I wanted or soaking up an informative podcast or just quietly reflecting, and considering I didn't mind the exercise, this was an agreeable enough situation. Until COVID hit. Initially we drivers were prepared to confront what for all intents and purposes seemed like another media-hyped health scare. We had worked through an Ebola scare and a Measles scare; COVID-19 wasn't about to hold up the hustle. And indeed it did not, although as blue-collar workers, we were outliers. As the economy shut down, and offices shuttered and people huddled in their homes through March, April, and May of 2020, we continued to work as if nothing had happened.

The experience of spending all day on the road during April of 2020 is something I doubt I'll ever forget. Traversing deserted streets alone began to make me feel like Will Smith in *I Am Legend*; every door I brought a twenty-four-pack of toilet paper or four cases of water to was potentially separating me from some person infected with the mysterious and nefarious virus. There was a pronounced general uncertainty in those days, and as shortages of basic supplies began to become a reality of day-to-day life, times became desperate. I remember once, before the arrival of industrial-scale orders of disinfection materials, pilfering an almost mint box of Clorox wipes from the lobby bathroom of a luxury apartment complex, my usual distaste for thievery momentarily overpowered by the necessity of sanitizing my workspace.

As I began to acclimate to "the new normal," making sure to tie my bandana around my face before work every day, using the company-provided disinfectant wipes to clean every single surface in the van's cab before entering, ignoring the hazmat workers stationed around the warehouse, the bleakness of my standing in the world began to set in. I had never been preoccupied with notions of social status or generational wealth, and so I had, on some level, come to accept what I perceived as a future in hard labor. Working with my hands, solving logistical problems, and relying on my spatial and situational awareness seemed like an agreeable lifestyle. The pandemic changed that and made me acutely aware of just how expendable our society views people like me. The patronizing way we were rebranded from "unskilled" to "essential" workers was a particularly insidious piece of propaganda, seemingly designed to allow us to hold on to a shred of our dignity as we braved a novel respiratory disease to deliver bored office workers dildos and video games.[1]

The day-to-day experience of showing up to work began to take on an increasingly surreal texture. Reminders to maintain social distance were plastered around the warehouse, and eventually such measures became literally built into the design of the facility as construction commenced on a maze of floor-to-ceiling industrial plastic dividers in the break room. In the warehouse where we loaded up in the mornings, management had deputized dozens of workers eager to get ahead of the hoard of pickers and packers, and who now relished any opportunity to display their loyalty by demanding drivers lift their mask to cover their nose or separating people with the six-foot stick they were uniformly issued by upper management as a tool for their work. Once we left the station, things were often just as strange and alien in the field, if not more. As a Black guy slowly and deliberately driving a white van through affluent suburbs, I was used to being ignored, and at times viewed with apprehensiveness, but being seen as a biohazard was certainly novel. As a matter of course, even from pre-pandemic times, I was already in the habit of generally making as little contact with customers as possible given their tendency of failing to grasp the nuances differentiating a "delivery person" from a "servant," but frequently upon seeing me approach their home, customers would come out and receive their package by hand anyway, shattering what meager pretense of social distance I had hoped to maintain. One customer came to the door wearing a sleep apnea mask, cord dangling down the front, and after seeing my exposed face chided me for my lax approach to my own personal safety. I chuckled and thanked him for his concern as I left, but he was not alone in his preoccupation with driver safety protocols. Touchdown management informed me of several people who filed complaints upon seeing me on their security cameras delivering a package to their residence while unmasked. The reality of being under constant surveillance was not new to me, but the degree to which customers felt agitated at my perceived lack of compliance was eye-opening, to say the least. Management assured me that they had waved away the complaints, aware, as I was, that if one were truly concerned with contaminated packaging, the lone last-mile delivery person was the least of their worries, but advised me to remain masked for all deliveries going forward lest the complaints form a pattern that corporate Amazon would have no choice but to address. Corporate Amazon, shining meritocracy that it is, for its part made token gestures of appreciation toward us in the form of "care packages," which generally were Ziplock bags with fun sized packs of cookies and potato chips, or, as on May Day 2020, a bottle of water and a pack of lemonade Crystal Light with a letter thanking us for "making lemonade out of lemons."

The guy who ran our operation, I'll call him Sean, had started out as a driver a few months before I had. Being almost double my age and brimming with type-A self-motivation, his status as a coworker of mine at our humble delivery company struck me as somewhat dissonant. There were rumors that he had retired from a successful career on Wall Street and took up blue collar cosplay in his late fifties for sport and exercise. His overbearing insistence that the rest of the staff adhere to whatever new obtuse doctrine corporate Amazon sent down the pipeline that week was annoying, but it also explained his rapid ascension from driver to dispatcher to shift manager to station manager. Noa, the Touchdown stakeholder who had established their franchise at Amazon Distribution Center NY 4, saw management material in Sean's monomaniacal drive to see 100% staff adherence to "the rules." Amazon paid Touchdown; Touchdown paid us; we should do what Amazon said, simple.

This would be dubious calculus under the best of circumstances and the outbreak of COVID-19 certainly was not that. Sean clearly maintained a sense of self by projecting adherence to structural norms; that these norms themselves may be detrimental to us, the workers, was of little concern to him. Amazon clearly had worked out this bountiful business model, why second-guess them in matters of logistical efficiency and personal safety? Noa, a fellow keen observer of human nature, understood Sean's contradictions, but as a business owner also understood that a manager so invested in employee conformity was invaluable to his bottom line.

Amazon DNY4 officially opened its doors in the summer of 2016, roughly a year and a half before I arrived. Formerly a Goya distribution hub, an Amazon spokesperson described the goal of the facility at the time to *Newsday* as "primarily serving customers in Nassau and Suffolk counties."[2] A little over a year into my time at the company, there were deliveries being shipped from that building to locations as far as the Bronx, South Brooklyn and even Westchester County. In 2015, the year before the facility opened, Amazon had reported net sales of $107 billion, putting it just behind the number-one retailer at the time, Walmart, which posted $478.6 billion in earnings the same year. Five years later, by the end of 2020, the first year of the COVID-19 pandemic, Amazon's yearly revenue was $386 billion, a hundred billion dollar increase from just the previous year.[3] This past August, Amazon finally dethroned Walmart to become the country's leading retailer, collecting $610 billion from consumers between June 2020 and June 2021, compared to Walmart's $566 billion in the same time span. There were roughly five to eight other Delivery Service Partner companies beside Touchdown in DNY4 while I worked there, all employing between fifty and one hundred people. According to the *Washington Post*, in November of 2020 Amazon had partnered with approximately seventeen hundred DSPs globally, and by October of this year that number was well over two thousand, according to *Vice*.[4,5] It's hard to overstate the voraciousness with which Amazon has rapidly consolidated not just the e-commerce space but ultimately retail overall, in New York, domestically in the United States, and globally. By the time I left, the company that seemed like a mysterious novelty to curious friends and family when I began working there in early 2018 had ascended to ominous ubiquity, largely propelled by the opportunity presented by the coronavirus and its effect on the economy.

At the onset of a once-in-a-lifetime pandemic, the notion of establishing a new baseline of acceptable workplace norms seemed ornately absurd, especially given the solitary nature of our work. As we lined up six feet away from one another one April morning, receiving our van keys and work devices from one of Sean's subordinate dispatchers who was almost too scared of the virus to make eye contact with us much less risk breathing the same air, I remember a fellow driver muttering to me on the way to his van, "Jesus, if you're scared to die, just stay home." If there was one thing we proved we were not, it was scared to die. Or at least, not so scared as to offset the demands of capitalism. And so we endured, unsure of whether the hundreds of boxes we handled a day, many from China, had COVID on their surfaces. Unsure exactly how much time it would take to catch the virus in close contact with warehouse workers as we loaded vans. If we're all moving in close quarters and breathing hard from exertion, how safe are these masks supposed to make us? I read online that only N95 masks protect against vapors; we're in a warehouse with hundreds of people wearing flimsy surgical masks, what's the point? Dispatchers would humor my queries with varying degrees of patience, but the ultimate answer remained the same: nobody knew, we were just following the protocol.

That tone of callous disingenuousness became prevalent working for Amazon during the pandemic. As demand for next-day home delivery of retail goods skyrocketed, the pressure on last-mile delivery drivers became more and more pronounced. Turnover was always high at Touchdown, but under those conditions people came and left at a more rapid rate than ever, putting a crunch on those of us that had made our peace with staying. On several occasions I came close to exchanging blows with other drivers and a few times even with management over miscommunications or perceived slights in the course of a workday. Ultimately violence was always avoided, and cooler heads prevailed, but there was a mutual understanding that we were all on edge and not of a mind to accept extraneous provocation. The stress of a higher workload amid the uncertainty of the moment was contrasted by the sunny, encouraging messaging our employer displayed not only internally but publicly as well, the urgency of customer satisfaction seemingly unable to be capitulated to fast enough. A coworker of mine who I was fond of, Adedayo, was tragically killed one morning after being ejected from the passenger seat of a Touchdown box truck on the 495. The driver, who had fallen asleep behind the wheel and rear-ended a flatbed truck, was saved from the same fate by the truck being mangled into a shape that cocooned him inside the cab on impact. These things happen. What strikes me now is how little acknowledgment there was of Adedayo and the accident at the time. The day it happened, I was one of the last drivers back to the station as Sean hurriedly rushed to the scene, his subordinate filling me in on the details as he drove off. Aside from a few hushed conversations in line to receive our van keys the next morning, that was essentially the last I heard of it. No vigil, no collection for his family, not even a moment of silence at morning meetup, so internalized was our collective subjugation that such company-wide gestures of humanity seemed frivolous and oxymoronic. We were there for one purpose only and there was no slack in the supply chain for grief.

Unsurprisingly (although also somewhat counterintuitively) Amazon's HR issues did come under some national scrutiny. In late March 2020, Chris Smalls, an assistant manager at an Amazon fulfillment center in Staten Island, was fired for what Amazon called "multiple safety violations." Smalls himself described his firing as "targeted retaliation" for helping to lead a protest against the company's lack of COVID preparations.[6] Smalls, who had worked at Amazon for five years at that point, claims to have witnessed the dissolving of his workplace's safety apparatus and instead of simply toeing the company line, demanded that his corporate overlords take action. Needless to say, Amazon wasn't going to bend to the whims of some ground-level assistant manager and instead of gearing up to address the glaring issues regarding workplace safety that were being brought to the fore, the company embarked on an acute campaign of character assassination to delegitimize Smalls and his message. While it would be an overstatement to say that they succeeded in that goal, the subtle messaging was still set firmly in place. Here was a young Black man, an individual deemed worthy of the management track in their company, now raising awareness of the callous nature of their business model; so their response was to describe him as "not smart or articulate" in "leaked" internal corporate memos and do their best to ignore the groundswell of support he quickly amassed, both within and outside of the community of Amazon workers and "essential" workers overall.[7]

I met Smalls at a May Day protest outside of Jeff Bezos's midtown Manhattan penthouse in 2021. He was demonstrating with a handful of associates from "The Congress of Essential Workers" (since rebranded as "The Amazon Labor Union"), a group made up of young to middle-aged men, mostly Black, several of whom worked under Chris during his tenure as an assistant manager. They were very willing to express their appreciation for Smalls not just as an outspoken leader against Amazon's campaign of exploitation, but also for his support and encouragement as a manager, making sure to convey that he routinely used his position of relative status within the company to help workers feel respected and appreciated. This young organization has gained support, both tactically and structurally, from individuals and groups long politically activated and invested in worker's rights as they have campaigned to unionize Amazon's labor force. After an unsuccessful 2021 election to unionize an Amazon facility in Bessemer, Alabama, was overturned due to the National Labor Relations Board's finding that Amazon improperly pressured staff to vote against the measure, there has been a potent resurgence of enthusiasm around the cause of unionization nationally and locally here in New York. Chris Smalls and the ALU, who traveled to Bessemer early last year to assist in the unionization effort, made themselves local fixtures at Staten Island warehouse facilities, holding barbecues and Q&A sessions in large tents stationed just outside the boundaries of Amazon property. To the acute dismay and embarrassment of the Amazon higher ups, the ALU helped workers at an Amazon facility in Staten Island known as JFK8 organize and win a union election—the first successful one at the company—2,654 to 2,131 in April 2022.[8]

It's been difficult to find the motivation to write this piece. My stint at Amazon is behind me now and were it not for my appreciation for a challenge, I may not even have gone through the motions of sifting through past trauma for the sake of "the historical record." That Amazon is a gargantuan economic force was a fact I was well aware of before beginning to work there in early 2018, but that ultimately made it all the more demoralizing to realize how little this company cared for its workers. In July 2021, Amazon founder Jeff Bezos, in a move recalling Gil Scott-Heron's classic poem "Whitey on the Moon," completed a suborbital joyride in the first manned flight of his private aerospace company Blue Origin. Blue Origin is less than transparent about its pricing structure, but according to CNBC, the top bid for a passenger seat on this maiden voyage was a cool $28 million.[9] Bezos is said to have invested at least $5.5 billion of his personal fortune in the company, which for a four-minute trip adds up to around $1.4 billion per minute. Upon landing, Bezos made sure to thank all Amazon employees for "paying for all this," which, frankly, I'm still unsure if he meant explicitly as an insult or not.[10] Regardless, the man and his ilk continue to rack up victories and "the little guy" is finding less and less room to maneuver between completely buying in to the global corporate vision for the world and total societal ostracization. While it has proven to be a massive boon for the company, this pandemic still is not over. Often it feels as if the state of it being "over" moves farther away into the horizon every day. And yet, somehow, the attendants of capital seem to be flourishing in spite of the pandemic, to the tune of $1.8 trillion in profit acquired by America's billionaires over the course of the pandemic, signaling to those of us who don't deem ambition a virtue that our lives will always matter less than those who strive at all costs.[11] I suppose as neoliberal subjects we've all been conditioned to crave some degree of hierarchical social stratification, something tangible to grasp onto to assure ourselves that we're better than somebody, anybody. I guess I'll just try to find a place to work that makes it a little less obvious.

Summer 2022

A few weeks ago I struck up a chat with an Amazon delivery driver I crossed paths with while working in Manhattan, asking him about his thoughts regarding the Amazon Labor Union. In my time since leaving Amazon I've found work as a driver for a nationally franchised moving company. This new job features virtually everything I liked about delivering for Amazon without the trademark Silicon Valley micromanagement, less crunch, less oversight, better tips. "Nah man, this is a temporary thing, I'm not really trying to be here that long" was his response when I probed to gauge his level of interest in joining the ALU. He was aware of Chris Smalls and his righteous crusade for worker's rights, but seemed unconvinced of the union's utility.

This ambivalence regarding the degree of influence the ALU is poised to wield was reflected in their election results on Staten Island. Although the union was victorious in their bid to unionize JFK8, the ALU's attempt to unionize sister Staten Island Amazon hub LDJ5, a sorting facility, was unsuc-cessful, with 618 employees voting against joining the union and 380 voting in favor.[12]

Overall, this reflects the broader context in which the ALU finds itself, where the American workers' movement is becoming more impassioned and more emboldened while also being met with the sort of strong resistance only a company as powerful as Amazon can facilitate. The ALU has organizing and actual administrative tasks to busy itself with, on top of such hindrances to progress as Amazon's strident resistance to negotiating and the notoriously brutal turnover rate for Amazon warehouse employees, which makes long-term employee investment in the union an even heavier lift. The necessity of the work is highlighted by the scale of the stakes against them, but for now, the ALU continues to fight.

CHAPTER 3

===

Double Jeopardy

Tania Darbouze

As soon as Governor Andrew Cuomo enacted a COVID-19 lockdown mandate in New York City, my family and I felt the brunt of the pandemic. Both of my parents are Haitian immigrants classified as "essential workers" who were in constant direct contact with the general public working in industries often dominated by Black immigrants. My father, who has always worked two jobs as an NYC school bus driver and an Access-A-Ride driver, was now faced with the reality that both of his jobs were up in the air due to the pandemic. For someone fortunate enough to have stable work for the previous two decades, this new uncertainty came as a shock. In our initial phone call after it was announced that things were shutting down, he told me he was uncertain when he would be able to go back to work, or if there would be any income coming in, caused instant anxiety on my end; because, whether he wanted to acknowledge it or not, I knew the very real realities of how thin our security blankets really were.

Like many other working-class or middle-class New Yorkers living essentially paycheck to paycheck, he was aware of the alarming reality that his survival was dependent on his labor. My father has worked constantly since he migrated from Haiti and has only called in sick once for an emergency appendix surgery. Even then, that was only after he completed his shift and drove himself to the hospital, where he was forced to take a couple of days off to recover. If that doesn't illustrate the lack of economic security and compassion in America for the working people, I don't know what does. My father didn't work two jobs, seven days a week, because he is a workaholic, but because he had the double responsibility of supporting our family in America and his family back home. So being laid off from work created double jeopardy not only in terms of survival for him, but also for his family back home who are still dependent on his financial support.

While facing financial insecurity, my father contracted COVID from a student on his bus and had a very touch-and-go recovery. During this time, he struggled with respiratory issues and general fatigue, which was a source of worry because he already had a preexisting condition and was in his sixties. After recovering from COVID, my father had to tackle acquiring unemployment benefits and because of the systematic failure across governmental departments to effectively address new unemployment issues, and the millions of New Yorkers trying to receive unemployment benefits, it took my father a few months to finally receive his benefits. Waiting to be onboarded was a stressful time because the state system was overwhelmed. It was a constant game of telephone and page refreshing, hoping to be the first on the call line. Because of this, his access to benefits was delayed and like many other Americans he didn't have years or even months of savings to fall back on.

My mother, on the other hand, faced a different reality when it came to the pandemic. She worked as a home health aide and was classified as an essential worker and was forced to continue to work during a global pandemic. Her employers used that classification to demand overtime hours from the workers without any time off. The home-health-aid industry is typically dominated by immigrant women who have sparse employment options and tend to stay within these industries as a means of survival. They are usually overworked, underpaid, and exploited. My mother is one of those women who didn't have the advantage of government mandates to protect her during the pandemic, giving her the ability to shelter at home and collect unemployment. Nor did she have a strong union that was focused on negotiating safer work conditions to prevent her from contracting the virus, being overworked, and exposing her to high patient-to-nurse ratios. Instead, she was pressured by her employers and was forced into working both her jobs back-to-back during a global pandemic. Her typical work routine during the pandemic consisted of using public transportation to commute to both jobs as a home health aide in a private home and a nursing home. She would work back-to-back shifts throughout the day and into the night, essentially working twenty-four hours straight. Her job consisted of providing direct care to the patients she worked with, and helping them maintain their everyday health and hygiene. Due to employers' pressures, a lack of governmental protection for essential workers, and the loss of workers who contracted the virus, she was denied paid time off and pressured into filling shifts for sick workers on her off days. This treatment went on until she got sick twice from sheer exhaustion and fatigue.

After working consistently from the beginning of the pandemic, my mother eventually contracted COVID, and as a result, my sister and I contracted COVID as well because we live with her and occasionally drive her to and from work. And although we live in a home that afforded us the luxury to quarantine separately that many New Yorkers do not have, we still contracted the virus from our mother. Getting access to proper medical care and COVID testing proved to be difficult because of the lack of accessible doctor offices in our neighborhood, scarce appointments, and the very strict rules doctor offices had during the pandemic. And because we were not confident in going to hospital emergency rooms, we turned to urgent care clinics instead. Urgent care clinics in our area were severely overwhelmed and had long lines that wrapped around the building and down the block. It took going to three separate urgent care offices before we were able to access a COVID test. But recovery for my mother was difficult and even after she recovered, she still had difficulty breathing, walking, and standing for a long period. Her new condition forced her into retiring early and cutting back her work shifts considerably. While my mother had significant savings to supplement her loss of income for a while, the situation created a new sense of worry if she would be able to provide for her family in New York City and her siblings back home.

While the media and government were praising frontline workers and calling them heroes, the COVID relief bills they brought to the table failed to protect America's working class. Their praise didn't provide hazard pay in the stimulus relief for front-line workers risking their health and their families. It didn't set limits and protections to create strategic work schedules where they would alternate shifts for nurses and home health aides working with the elderly to prevent burnout. It is clear that the government considers the labor of the American people more important than their lives, their families, and their survival.

COVID set ablaze the realization that the American infrastructure is deadly to the American people and especially deadly to Black people. COVID-19's racial implications are due to preexisting and historic racial disparities in housing, health care, generational wealth/household income, employment opportunities, and social mobility. So when the media and other sources indicate that Black people are dying at a much higher rate than other groups of people, what is missing from the context are the social and environmental conditions we are forced to live under that contribute to the rising Black death tolls. Without foregrounding sociopolitical conditions in the discussion of the pandemic, Black death tolls almost seem coincidental or situational or, even worse, due to the flawed bodies of Black people rather than deliberate cause and effect. This pandemic has highlighted how much systematic racism affecting Black people in America has been camouflaged as "essential work" and "normal" everyday urban settings. It is these urban settings that have made the virus a super spreader in neighborhoods like East Flatbush, Canarsie, Bed-Stuy, Greenpoint, and Coney Island. In neighborhoods like these, the sheer density of people living alongside one another and in surrounding apartments makes it difficult to prevent the spread of the virus. Due to economic strains, lack of generational wealth, ethnic cultural norms, and the high cost of living, people in these communities often live in houses and apartments with more people than there are rooms, so there is no possibility of social distancing or proper quarantining. If someone is affected by the virus it is easily spread throughout the household and the community. According to research dating from the height of the pandemic, "In every age category, Black people are dying from COVID at roughly the same rate as white people a decade older." Black people, no matter what age, were dying rapidly because of their susceptibility to greater workplace exposures.[1] My family and many other Black New York City residents did not have the ability to work from home, to take sick days, or have the financial ability to flee NYC and move into the suburbs.

With virtually no safety net of savings, many Black residents in NYC have had to weigh out the risk of exposure or not going to work and losing their livelihoods and ability to support their households. Inadequate health care is also a factor in the outcome of COVID in Black neighborhoods because there is less access to COVID-19 testing, health professionals, and facilities that can meet the demands of a higher number of patients. Black people are already susceptible to preexisting health conditions such as blood pressure, hypertension, and asthma due to environmental racism and lack of healthier food options.[2] These preexisting health conditions, when met with the coronavirus, make for bigger complications where it is harder to survive the disease. All of these preexisting conditions played a huge factor in Black death tolls in New York City. Even though Black residents only make up

12.5% of our population, they accounted for 22.6% of all deaths to COVID-19 in the early months of the pandemic. In the first phase of the pandemic, Black people in New York City were also two times as likely to die from coronavirus than white people, and two times as likely to be hospitalized for nonfatal COVID-19 cases.[3] In 2022, death toll rates varied up and down for different ethnic groups. Later data showed that Black deaths scaled back and that the white population accounted for higher death tolls. Because the white population is older than populations of color, and COVID-19 mortality rates have been higher among older people, these unadjusted estimates are likely to underestimate racial inequalities, particularly for COVID-19 deaths.[4]

Missing from the conversation about how the pandemic has been deadlier and more consequential for Black people in NYC is the double jeopardy many Black immigrants face in the pandemic. For many immigrants who carry the double burden of providing for both their family in the United States and back home, any lost income affects the whole family. The struggle for survival is even more intense when you have family members in your countries of origin who depend on you for schooling, and basic necessities like food, shelter, and access to health care. Black immigrants who live in NYC make up the largest ethnic/racial group of front-line workers in transportation, health care, and grocery store jobs, which made them more susceptible to catching the virus and dying from COVID. Black workers represent more than 40% of transportation workers in NYC; 32% of workers in childcare, family, homeless, and food services; and 33% of truckers and postal workers.[5] In addition to being part of an unequal, segregated labor force, Black immigrants usually don't have the luxury of working remotely; instead, they must work outside every day serving the public. Even more devastating is that during a global pandemic ICE raids continued across NYC but specifically in neighborhoods like East Flatbush, Bed-Stuy, and Crown Heights, where there are large populations of Black immigrants, forcing many of them to close down their businesses and shops in fear of deportation. Brooklyn neighborhoods like East Flatbush became a ghost town where African beauty shops, Haitian bakeries, Dominican restaurants, and local vendors and laborers all closed shop to help prevent themselves and their employees from being deported.

Since the beginning of the pandemic both my parents have been trying to focus on recouping lost income from the pandemic and dealing with the lingering health implications of COVID. While my father has been able to supplement some lost income with unemployment, and a percentage of money his union was able to negotiate for workers at his job, my mother is still trying to figure out how she will manage. Retired from working in private home health care, she is now trying to adjust financially from two incomes to one. This financial change has been drastic for us as a family because she didn't expect to retire this early without having a thorough backup plan. She is able to make ends meet, but only because she consistently dips into her savings. This puts more pressure on us as her kids to work to supplement some of that lost income and maintain our household. This drastic shift has been a challenge for her to adjust to because she is no longer in the same place physically or financially that she was just a year or two ago. Healthwise, she has been dealing with brain fog, constant fatigue, and muscle spasms—all after-effects of contracting COVID at her place of employment. Since the pandemic and graduating college, I have started working two jobs in order to try and relieve some of the economic burden on my parents.

The government has prioritized big corporations and massive tax breaks when providing COVID relief packages while debating if American working-class people need additional COVID relief aside from two underwhelming stimulus checks. When we see how other countries are handling this pandemic and providing monthly, consistent financial support, strict lockdowns, free medical care, and other needed support, it is clear that the inaction of elected officials is deliberate and calculated. Americans have had to resort to mutual aid funds, GoFundMes, and community drives to support one another when we should have had governmental support. There is no telling when the pandemic will end but we as a nation will never be able to go back to life pre-pandemic. While we have lost thousands of Black lives to the virus here in NYC, the Black unemployment rate doubled early in the pandemic, and thousands of people were displaced and evicted for not being able to pay rent.[6] The economic fallout has affected the Black community the most, and legislation should focus on making sure that relief does more than trickle down to disenfranchised communities and front-line workers.

CHAPTER 4

Beloved, but Forced to Live
and Die in the Shadows

Yamilka Portorreal

April 10, 2020, marked less than one week until my twenty-first birthday. I was excited to hit this milestone despite the onset of the COVID-19 pandemic. I had accepted that I would not be able to celebrate it the way I always wanted to: with a lot of friends. However, I was very grateful that everyone in my immediate family was okay and no one had contracted COVID yet. That afternoon, my grandmother was making coffee when she got a call from an old friend. In hindsight, I was too focused on my chemistry homework to really notice her boisterous shock and confusion. I thought one of her distant family members whom I'd never met before had passed away, which is usually the case, but this time it felt different. Her surprise was accompanied by crying.

"He died?!!!" she exclaimed in Spanish.

As soon as she hung up the phone, she headed in my direction in what felt like light speed. I vividly remember the smell of roasted coffee beans that followed her as she entered my room.

"What happened?" I said obliviously.

"Leo died!" she exclaimed, as she burst into tears.

I felt my heart drop. I was bombarded with feelings of shock, confusion, sadness, and a multitude of questions.

"How could it have been possible?! I trusted that he would get better," I thought to myself.

Our suspicion of coronavirus was true. Since tests weren't widely available in April, we had to assume that Leonardo was sick from COVID-19 based on his symptoms of fever and cough. He was also undocumented, which made it challenging for him to seek medical help. It is likely he never pursued medical assistance for fear of deportation, a dilemma many undocumented people face. A literature review of PubMed's publications illustrates that fear of deportation was a prominent barrier to health care access in 65% of the articles analyzed; 36% of articles indicated that an inability to communicate in English was also a barrier.[1] In other words, fear of deportation is an overwhelming concern among undocumented immigrants, and it comes with little trust for the health care system. This prevents them from accessing proper health care and forces them to rely on home remedies and over-the-counter medicine to alleviate their ailments. Undocumented people have been systematically denied access to a basic service that is necessary for the survival of the pandemic: health care.

"Would his fate have been different if he had received medical help on time?" I asked myself, as my eyes filled with tears.

"Maria told me that he was getting better," my grandma said, "but he started coughing up blood and died shortly after, alone in his room. His roommate (who also presumably contracted COVID-19) found him after it had happened."

We cried as we shared many memories we had of him. The next few weeks passed, and I was still in denial. It was easy to be in this state because there was no funeral, no physical evidence, just a call. I spent my birthday grieving his death. As time went on, I realized that I had no choice but to accept it. I constantly thought about how the circumstances robbed him of any humanity.

Life before the World Turned Upside Down

I migrated from the Dominican Republic to the United States in 2009 at ten years of age. My grandmother was the first person in our family to migrate here, followed by my father and me. He needed some time to get settled before he could bring the rest of my family, so he rented an apartment in the Bronx where we lived together for a little while.

My grandmother became my caregiver. She made a living as a street vendor in Washington Heights selling Dominican flour patties called *pastelitos*, and cassava-based patties called *empanadas de yuca*. Her cart was conveniently placed a few blocks away from my middle school, which meant that once school ended, I had to stay in the street while she finished working for the day. I tried to help her any way I could, whether it was running errands or pushing her cart into storage for the next day.

My grandmother became a street vendor because it required no formal education and she was able to work for herself. When she started out, she received guidance from another more experienced and well-known street vendor in the neighborhood nicknamed *la vecina*, or the neighbor. On the same block, there was a Jewish-owned-but-immigrant-run clothing store staffed by Dominican and Mexican workers. It was one of the owner's two locations in Washington Heights. Throughout the years, the workers grew very fond of my grandmother and treated us like family. Maria, Leonardo, and Ana used to run the store. Ana was the cashier because she could speak a little bit of English, while Maria and Leonardo did everything else. (Their names have been changed to protect their identities.)

Leonardo was selfless and loyal, and he liked to joke around. Many people in the neighborhood became very fond of him, and he became like a second father figure to me. When it was too cold out, he would sometimes offer me hot chocolate, one of his favorite drinks. At times, he was very observant and quiet, it seemed as though his mind was somewhere else. Ana and Maria were also very welcoming and supportive, always making sure that we were okay. I remember that for Christmas 2010, I wanted to get a video game, but my dad could not afford it, so they all saved up some of their money to buy me that gift. I was so happy and thankful that they had gone above and beyond to make me feel like family. I will always be grateful to them for everything they have done for us.

Leonardo didn't share a lot of details about his past because it caused him a lot of pain. I learned he was raised in Mexico by his grandparents because his parents had abandoned him. I had to piece his past together based on what my grandmother told me. In a way, we became his family. Our chosen family was not particular to Leonardo. It's a means of survival for immigrants because it provides community care through the daily relationships they cultivate with fellow community members, and Leo was beloved by his community. It was not unusual to see him waving hello to people who were passing by, sharing jokes with the regulars that came to the store to hangout.

Community care is very important to immigrants, especially undocumented people, who lack access to many basic rights and services. During the pandemic, one example of this was the rise in mutual aid. Mutual aid is the exchange of vital resources between community members through the distribution of food and relief funds for those who are most in need when the state fails to provide people's necessities. For example, early in the pandemic, the co-founders of the Washington Heights nonprofit Uplift needed drivers to disperse food donations throughout the community; there's such a tight-knit community that local grassroots volunteers decided to do the job while placing themselves at risk for catching the virus.[2] The drivers were willing to place themselves at a greater risk to feed those in the community who lack resources and were food insecure, including undocumented people. The absence of resources shows how marginalized undocumented people are; mutual aid highlights the importance of community care to marginalized people: because they cannot rely on the government to provide for them in times of crisis, they rely on each other.

Community care was present in Leo's housing. The status of undocumented people makes it difficult for them to be able to rent an apartment. However, since Leo was so well-connected in the community, he was able to rent a room near his worksite in the apartment of another community member. He lived there for more than five years, until his tragic death.

Leo decided to come to the United States to find a better life, so he crossed the US-Mexico border in the late 1980s and ended up in New York, where he started working at a tailor shop in downtown Manhattan. Later he found a job at the store on 178th and that's where he stayed all this time, never having a spouse or children. Like many undocumented people, he dedicated his life to working in the United States, and the pandemic showed that no matter how much of their life they have devoted to this country, they are not going to receive the same treatment as documented folks, evidenced in the lack of financial resources and medical assistance. Not having access to either of those can be catastrophic, and the lack of security increased during the pandemic.

I graduated middle school in 2012, and my mother and sister came to the United States shortly after. My grandmother went back to D.R. for a few years while I started going to high school in Harlem. My grandmother's absence meant that I had no active link to the life I had built in Washington Heights.

During my high school career, a lot of my middle school friends had to move elsewhere due to increasing rents brought about by the gentrification of Washington Heights. Ana decided to quit her job as a cashier at the store, so Maria and Leonardo were left with all the work. Finally, the rent was so high that the owner was obligated to close the 178th Street location. Leonardo and

Maria were transferred to work at his other store. The fabric of community was being destroyed by the displacement of its residents.

Chaos

When I was a senior at Brooklyn College, my grandma decided to stay with us for one of her US trips. We had agreed that we were going to visit Leonardo and Maria when the time was right, but unfortunately, that never happened. I was struggling a lot with balancing school and work, and at times, the stress was too much to handle. My everyday one-and-a-half-hour commute from the Bronx to Brooklyn did not make it any better. We were patiently waiting for my next break to meet up, but shortly after, the pandemic started.

Leonardo was working at the clothing store before the governor's executive order on March 20 to shut down nonessential businesses. That's likely how he contracted COVID-19. Although he was not an essential worker, an overwhelming majority of undocumented workers are. One study estimates that more than two-thirds of undocumented workers are essential workers.[3] Like all essential workers, they were not being compensated in any form for their increased risk because there is no hazard pay. Of the 1.2 million jobs lost in New York City due to the pandemic, 192,000 are estimated to be jobs held by undocumented immigrant workers.[4] Undocumented workers were also twice as likely to lose their jobs in other parts of the nonessential service industry.

Already in a position with few options to ask for assistance, the loss of employment can be devastating. During the COVID-19 pandemic, access to unemployment could mean the difference between life and death. The Coronavirus Aid Relief and Economic Security Act (CARES) benefits were denied to families even if only a single person in the family was undocumented.[5] The government used guilt by association to deny people their benefits. It is cruel that you can be a tax-paying undocumented worker, yet the government does not guarantee you or your family any protection during times of crisis, even if you are entitled to that compensation.

Maria shared Leo's roommates' account of his death. People in hazmat suits picked up his body in an ambulance, and since he had no next of kin, his body was labeled as *unclaimed*. The city took responsibility for his burial—likely in the isolated spot where the city buries the unhoused, the sick, the unclaimed, and the poor: Hart Island. Although Leonardo was present in our lives, the community, and the workforce of this country, the circumstances of the pandemic made his passing invisible.

Many New Yorkers are unaware of Hart Island, a public cemetery located off the eastern coast of the Bronx. The city purchased Hart Island in 1868, and since then, it has been used to bury the unclaimed, stillborn, soldiers, the unhoused, victims of the HIV/AIDS epidemic and poor people.[6] It has been a place where those who are marginalized are buried. Hart Island has also been used to house various institutions such as a tuberculosis hospital, a quarantine station for people with yellow fever, an insane asylum, a jail, a missile base, a narcotic rehabilitation program and a military base.[7] Hart Island has not been immune to the effects of the pandemic either. According to city data, three thousand out of the first thirty thousand people who died of COVID-19 in New York City were buried on Hart Island, a significant increase from the 846 bodies buried there in 2019.[8] The city reached a point where it was so inundated with dead bodies that the government could not keep up with contacting relatives.[9] There is a good possibility that Leonardo was buried on Hart Island, since he died so early in the pandemic, which coincided with the timeline when the city was overwhelmed by bodies.

Leonardo's story provides a human dimension behind the statistics. At the end of the day, he was more than just a number, and his death had ripple effects in the community. It seems so contradictory that he was so visible during life, yet so invisible during death.

My story is intertwined with my immigration, a chosen family, street vending, gentrification, and Leo's story. His story reflected his visibility and importance in the community, yet his status as an undocumented immigrant rendered him disposable by the same economic and social system he had served most of his life. Although the pandemic made his death invisible and quiet, the loss of his radiant and caring presence couldn't have been more noticeable. He was truly an asset to the people around him. It is unsettling to imagine that he may have hesitated to seek out life-saving medical treatment because of his undocumented status. Lack of health care and other safety nets were catastrophic during the pandemic, especially for undocumented people. Leo was more than a statistic. Like many other undocumented immigrants, he represented more than his contributions of to the workforce, he repre-sented an integral person in Washington Heights who helped hold the com-munity together. He was a kid who grew up in Mexico with his grandparents and came to the United States to work for a lifetime, but most importantly, he made a mark as an essential part of a community that will persist after his tragic death. Undocumented people contribute to the economy and their communities, building a chosen family away from their native countries, which helps them and this city be more resilient. Yet no matter how essential and visible they are in their communities, in the eyes of American institutions, they are obligated to live in the shadows. Telling Leo's story and acknowledging the important roles of undocumented people throughout American society counteracts the silence that allows their oppression to continue.

CHAPTER 5

When Essential Student Workers Strike Back

Alan Aja

September 2020: As soon as the last student logs off from class, I close the sylla-bus and presentation tabs, run to refill my cup of coffee, and jump back in my seat to open the meeting link and agenda. Much like our students, participants log in from across each city's many neighborhood enclaves, although in this case some join in from their suburban or out-of-state homes. The backdrops vary as cameras turn on—some colleagues are in their home offices, an actual room dedicated to their work they may share with family, others are in their living room, kitchen, bedroom, or whatever make-shift space they can create for work. Brooklyn College's department chairs and program directors, ranging in age, academic rank, and economic status, meet in respective isolation not just in the context of fear and uncertainty as the virus continues to rip through the city, but also to consider the economic health of their departments and institution.

It wasn't supposed to be this kind of meeting. After finishing the second semester of a sabbatical, I returned to the emotional weight of chairing one of the few remaining ethnic studies departments in the country with "Puerto Rican Studies" in its title and central curricular focus. Born out of student organizing and activism during the early 1970s wave of "ethnic revival," the academic unit, now in its fifty-second year, has withstood larger historical forces in the US academy of disciplinary redundancy or closure, mergers with other area or ethnic studies and/or conversion to a lesser-resourced program.[1] These forces, however, didn't exist in a vacuum, and there was a cruel irony in this particular cyber-meeting as colleagues discussed not the typical admin-istrative mundanities, but fears for their respective academic units of what was the pre-pandemic norm of treatment for ethnic studies writ large. "Historically, human made calamaties have often served as cover for drastic cuts to public higher education. We feared that the pandemic would create a pretext for such cuts at CUNY."² Just a few months earlier, administrators had already begun unnecessary austerity measures, citing expected inadequate state revenues as a result of lower student enrollments during the pandemic. In this meeting, chairs and program directors discussed their fears of the new reality—cuts to course sections, increasing class sizes (at this point now fully online), non-reappointed adjuncts, fewer incoming resources to our academic units, and most frightening, the prospect of departmental "closure" or "restructuring."³ At one point, sensing that we were being "divided and conquered" per austerity's design, one of my colleagues stated openly that in order to save more "important" departments, they could see us, and other small, interdisciplinary studies units, as expendable amid the fiscal morass.

In this early pandemic moment, with what felt like the department's future seemingly on the line, all I could think of is "not on our students' backs, and not on my watch." It wasn't long into the subsequent academic year, as campus leadership pushed full steam ahead into austerity mode, that the intersection of the George Floyd uprisings and the pandemic would place reignited spotlights on higher education's racist institutional structures and practices—the storied Brooklyn College being no exception. At a summer 2021 rally held at a college entrance and co-organized by our faculty and staff union, held both in person and streamed online, one by one, speakers representing students, staff, faculty, and alumni called for a new structural vision and reality for their beloved institution. Demands would include the release of stimulus monies presently withheld by the administration toward an anti-racist plan that centered increased health and safety measures, reduced class sizes, restored adjunct positions, funded ethnic studies departments, and remedies for the paucity of Black, Latinx, Asian, and Indigenous faculty.⁴ During a nervous bull-horn speech of my own, I pointed to the surrounding spiked gates of the college as symbolic of the intra-institutional barriers CUNY's working-class students of color persistently face. Afterward, activists from the Puerto Rican Alliance (PRA), MEDo (Movimiento Estudiantil Dominicano), and other student clubs, the former being the very historic student organization that over half a decade ago was instrumental in the formation of the department, surrounded me and each other with supportive words.

"We got each others' backs, Profe."

"Estaremos listos (we'll be ready) to organize if they (administrators) don't listen."

"We're forming an action committee and meeting soon with the alum to make a plan."

"En la lucha (in the struggle)!"

In the midst of a deadly pandemic, where CUNY students are ready to defend their intellectual homes even as they work multiple jobs and their economic and family lives are forever disrupted, their awe-inspiring words and action seem foretelling of the possible yet to come.

The Essentiality of (Student) Work

Amid another seemingly endless wave of COVID-19 infection, this one due largely to the B5 variant, the *Intercept* published a well-circulated piece exposing a Bank of America internal memo's "hope" that increasing worker power would dissipate.[5] As the pandemic unfolded and laid bare longtime structural inequities (while those inequities themselves deepened the pandemic), workers in the most vulnerable industries began to push back, demanding higher wages and increased health and safety workplace protections. That a financial giant, already raking in excess profits during the pandemic's rising inflation, would want workers to lose ground isn't a surprise—by capitalism's longtime design, banks profit neatly off abrupt "shocks" in the economy when workers are vulnerable and have less power over their work lives.[6]

When we consider the autoethnographies in *Until We Are Seen*, particularly how Samantha Saint Jour, Zayd Brewer, Tania Darbouze, Yamilka Portorreal, and others expose the hidden underbellies of "essential work" they undertake as they support their families and balance their education, what is "seen" is exactly what the banks and ruling class writ large are worried about. These student writers not only debunk the neoliberal economic theories that inform the public policies and media coverage that affect their lives, but also provide a window onto the current and future trajectory of workers exerting their class consciousness.[7]

As Theoharis and Entin note in the introduction, while a predominant view of the college experience is one of residential campuses where recent high school graduates concentrate on their studies over an expected period of four years, the typical college experience (85%) in the United States is that of commuter students whose lives are entangled with family responsibilities and work necessary to fund their education.[8] A recent AAUP report on "working college students" revealed that, to manage exponentially increasing college costs and dwindling student aid, an overwhelming number of undergraduate students work more than twenty hours a week. This is especially true for low-income students of color at under-resourced institutions like CUNY and CSULA.[9]

That the necessity of student work is consistently detached from prevailing narratives about higher education in the United States isn't an accident. The fiscal assault on public higher education since the 1980s, when low-income people and people of color began accessing it in higher numbers, is a negative reaction to the possibility of an educated and empowered working class. In my nearly two decades at CUNY, this fiscal violence has been abundantly clear, whether from teaching in a chronically under-resourced, historic ethnic studies department that helps prepare future graduate students and bilingual educators or in codirecting a research program for transfer students that relies on foundation support for its existence.[10] Even when everyone from faculty to administrators to elected officials readily admit that CUNY students deserve radically more fiscal support, acknowledging the family economies that rely on their labor and celebrating them as "resilient" and "heroes" during the pandemic, the burden (if not blame) is on working students to maneuver around the repressive structural conditions that shape their educational lives. Never mind that the state and the institution have a moral mandate to provide a well-funded, high-quality education.

Before we consider how these student writers refuse to accept these conditions, or "strike back," to use an empowered work analogy, let me first set the theoretical context that predominates policymaking in higher education.[11] The infamous "human capital theory" of mainstream economics posits that individuals forego earnings, building their credentials through higher education in order to achieve a wage that over the long run supposedly makes up for that initially deferred income. Notwithstanding that "payoffs" for education are unequal across social groups, especially for younger workers of color, or that this can beget the debilitating load of student debt, what's important here is the assertion that any material (wage) difference experienced from that point is on the individual (and/or the social group they belong to).[12] The reasons for any "gaps" are myriad, but often reduced to the behavioral—a supposed result of the individual's lack of education, skills, effort, motivation, or cultural values.[13] Relatedly, from the never-ceasing "culture of poverty" theories, individuals, (read: people of color) are blamed for any adverse educational or labor market disparities they face—a supposed result from their own destructive and counteractive behaviors passed down across generations. The autoethnographies here upend these deficit-based narratives by default—and in an ideal world, would put these racist theories to rest once and for all.

Take, for instance, the strong critiques and contradictions of "essential worker" the autoethnographies present so vividly, beginning with the intersecting analyses Samantha Saint Jour and Zayd Brewer each lay out for readers. Samantha, when cursed out by a mask-refuser at her McDonald's job, the very work she needed to support her education, writes that her hostile treatment "definitely reminded me that even though minimum-wage workers are 'essential workers,' working through the pandemic to provide food and supplies, we will never be treated as essential. . . . Our importance is constantly overlooked, even when we're the last ones providing necessities." Zayd likewise calls out the hypocrisy of pandemic rhetoric: "The patronizing way we were rebranded from 'unskilled' to 'essential' workers was a particularly insidious piece of propaganda seemingly designed to allow us to hold on to a shred of our dignity as we braved a novel respiratory disease to deliver bored office workers dildos and video games."

Zayd and Samantha indeed unveil something insidious here that deserves attention. Re-labeling once supposedly stigmatized "unskilled" work as "essential" provided semantic cover for a vast array of dangerous and underpaid work under the guise of heroic and crucial service for the life of the economy. As background, a recent study by the Fiscal Policy Institute revealed that "essential workers" are disproportionately women, immigrant, Black and Latinx, far more likely to live under the poverty line, and labor in service and other lower-paying sectors.[14] Like some of our student-autoethnographers in this book, they work in public transit, delivery, and warehouse industries; bodegas (convenience stores), food industries, and supermarkets; and childcare and health care facilities, among other locations. Yet, as the Economic Policy Institute finds in their own report, essential workers don't have access to the most basic workplace health and safety protections, increasing the likelihood of sickness and death.[15] Both reports underscore the "essential" group's disturbing wage exploitation.

To put the above differently, while Zayd, Samantha, and others help us learn more about workers' conditions *within-pandemic*, they also lay bare the historical obfuscation and residual effects of the *pre-pandemic*. Prior to the notorious spring of 2020, unemployment and underemployment in "precarious" (unstable, low-paid, often unsafe, and nonunion) work were already the growing norm for workers of color.[16] It wasn't long ago that reckless financial transactions through deregulated capitalism gave us the "Great Recession," widening already racialized income and wealth gaps to unconscionable levels amid ongoing evisceration of crucial safety nets.[17] Over a decade later, the so-called "Great Resignation" projected an image of workers tired by pandemic-related struggles, using their agency and leverage as they sought better opportunities. Never mind that for many essential workers, this agency was limited by long-baked hostile workplace conditions and union busting obfuscated from the public narrative. As the pandemic unfolded, report after report compared any improvements for workers to "pre-pandemic levels"; these analyses simultaneously erased the humanity of workers who died or were exposed to long-term effects of the virus and tended to normalize long-standing workplace and other material inequities.[18]

The "Globality" of Essential (Exploited) Work

The conditions workers faced in Los Angeles and New York during the pandemic cannot be separated from the disproportionate impact of COVID on these two cities: the former had the highest death rate in the nation, and the latter the second-highest. Anthony Almojera (see Chapter 11) knows this firsthand—a twenty-year veteran in arguably the most "front-line" work of the pandemic, Emergency Medical Services (EMS), he applies the military analogy of "collateral damage" as a lucid and appropriate descriptive of the "sick society we respond to." Placing the racialized inequities of his job (the irony of less sick leave and disproportionate economic precarity emergency responders face) in the larger context of a market-based health care system and the struggles for (supposedly) scarce resources that public workers face, his testimony strikes back at the famed "global city" model. If particular cities would serve as central nodes of interconnected global production that attract capital and labor and hence supposedly transfer wealth across groups and improve living conditions, Anthony forces us to ask the too-often-omitted basic questions of "whose labor?" and exactly "what capital?"

As a further example of the consequences of this predominant economic model, let us consider the hidden material underbellies of the famed "ethnic enclaves" where many of our student writers reside. Neighborhoods where food, cultural diversity, and artistic expression are often celebrated, these are the same segregated sites of economic production where immigrants were expected to sacrifice, through labor immobility and exploitation, for subsequent generations' eventual "assimilation" into the economically stable mainstream. Once the prevailing discourse, these longtime theories speak more to an early to mid-twentieth-century white ethnic immigrant experience where government and institutional support was key in building intergenerational wealth to assure this economic mobility.[19] Most of today's ethnic enclaves, absent the same historic government investment as yesteryear's migrants had, are marked instead by the prevalence of nonunion, low-paid, unstable work that rely on exploited local and migrant (often undocumented) labor. Thus, for immigrant children specifically—absent yesteryear's government support and education viewed as the primary "way out" of the exploitative enclave conditions—their parents must make the ultimate sacrifice.

Yamilka Portorreal's illuminating and powerful autoethnography helps us understand these "trade-off" expectations. Describing her family's economic struggles in the longtime resource-poor and spatially segregated Dominican ethnic enclave of Washington Heights, she contextualizes the forces of gentrification and displacement that positioned her family, and specifically her family friend Leo (may he rest in peace), as a labor migrant within his own city. That an undocumented immigrant is unable to seek medical help for fear of deportation (while relying on home remedies), serves as a harrowing referendum on the US immigration and health care apparatus as well as a larger capitalist system that relies on vulnerable laborers while denying them the most basic human rights.

The same goes for Tania Darbouze's parents. Both immigrants from Haiti and working in local industries ("ethnic niches") long dominated by Black immigrants through immigration-work recruitment policies, she demonstrates how a "family economy" could collapse at the pandemic's appearance. On the one hand, her mother was thrust into the category of essential worker, given her job as a home health care aide, with the irony of guaranteed employment in long, harrowing, dangerously virus-exposed shifts where workers were already notoriously "overworked, underpaid, and exploited." Her father was also directly subjected to the virus's harm. "Like many other working-class or middle-class New Yorkers living essentially paycheck to paycheck, he was aware of the alarming reality that his survival was dependent on his labor." Tania underscores how his health, like her mom's experiences in a poorly health-regulated industry, came second to work, stating that he "didn't work two jobs seven days a week because he is a workaholic." She also references the typical "double responsibility" and "double-jeopardy" of transnational migrants, in which workers are financially responsible for themselves and their families abroad through remittances.[20]

How We "Strike" Back

Tania, Anthony, Samantha, and others allow us to look outside the statistics to value their families' lives, countering the ways essential work renders people as invisible cogs in the capitalist wheel. They also provide critical insight that could inform social movements to bold, transformative policies. For instance, Samantha eviscerates the role of the state in perpetuating intergroup inequities through its inadequate pandemic response ("no solutions were presented, just hollow words of appreciation for our leaders"), and she is ahead of the game policy-wise. She points out that part-time work is not sustainable; in rightfully criticizing the federal pandemic response by Congress and the Biden administration, she distinguishes the material difference between conservative, incrementalist policy proposals (read: establishing a federal minimum wage of $15) and material-level practice (read: the egregious economic inadequacy of said wage). While we are still a long way from a $15 federal minimum wage, Samantha instead points to the crucial need for a "living wage," which, in considering the localized cost of living and inflation, calculates to much higher than any state or local minimum. She underscores that the same groups (young people, women, people of color) affected by poverty and exploitation are also "the same groups being disproportionately affected by the pandemic in other ways, such as mental illness, domestic violence, unemployment, and police brutality."

Undoubtedly, while Samantha's foresight intersects with the many autoethnographies in this book that contextualize their authors' experiences amid a dwindling safety net, Zayd's wit provides an additional window onto the state's corporate enablers (and through subsidies and tax breaks, its actual beneficiaries). In highlighting how his employer, Amazon, "the shining meritocracy that it is," created care packages of Ziplock bags full of "fun-sized" treats and offered packs of lemonade Crystal Light with a letter of thanks for "making lemonade out of lemons," he unveils perhaps the most absurd and egregious metaphor of the pandemic: thanks for your labor, here's a doggy bag. When workers struck back through union organizing, Zayd highlighted the grotesque pushback from the company—tactics long used by the ruling class and their anointed managers to retain power structures, a response that acknowledges worker power as a threat to corporate rule.

The pieces reinforce the effectiveness of workers confronting capital directly. There's growing evidence that during the pandemic, "essential" workers across industries have made gains in forming more unions and acquiring health care insurance, workplace protections, pay raises, paid sick leave, and other necessities.[21] At the time of writing, workers from the aisles of Trader Joe's to the distribution warehouses of Amazon to the registers of Starbucks to the railyards of Appalachia to the floors of the most well-resourced hospitals and beyond represent perhaps a reignited pan-generational revolt for basic economic rights. Workers, from baristas to nurses, have clearly struck back. In addition, in line with these movements, there are also urgent calls here by our writers for universal public goods. Much of my own research and scholarly trajectory has also underlined how government should work "for all" through guaranteed housing, health care, jobs, income, care work, transportation, and education. But in order to do that equitably, society's most vulnerable must be centered in everything from policy design to implementation.

The autoethnographies also make claims for horizontal systems of support through "everyday revolutions."[22] Not necessarily the larger-scale movements romanticized in historical ether, they advocate for community-level approaches through cooperative aid and later organizing that to improve the immediate social and environmental condition as new systems are imagined and constructed. We return to Yamilka and Daniel (Sanabria—see Chapter 16) respectively, who offer the alternative of "mutual aid," as Yamilka nicely defines it, as "the exchange of vital resources between community members through the distribution of food and relief funds for those who are most in need when the state fails to meet people's necessities." Yamilka's example of drivers organized by a local community nonprofit to distribute food to insecure people, regardless of immigration status, is a powerful (and evidently dangerous and unsustainable) way of striking back when the state fails to deliver. In the colonial, neglected context of Puerto Rico, Daniel highlights a "praxis of care," as he centers his sister who engaged in mutual aid by producing and selling masks.

In the end, both examples are powerful indictments of state abandonment and the need for structural policy change to ensure the health and safety of all. They provide radical models for the future of work, ones that, whether informal or formal, vertical or horizontal, brick-and-mortar or cyberspace, diapora or island, abandon no one and protect everyone.

PART II

Racism, Family, and Commitments
in a Time of Emergency

CHAPTER 6

Me, My Mom, and Her Mental Illness

Billie-Rae Johnson

My mom has had schizophrenia my whole life and got it while serving in the army. I am an only child. My parents divorced when I was young. We're estranged from our other family members because there is a lot of stigma around my mom having a mental illness. Furthermore, my mom doesn't have a partner, and she's very antisocial so I'm her main source of social interaction.

Life Before the Pandemic

I'm ten in the fifth grade. We've been staying with my grandma for two weeks. She lives in an independent housing development for senior citizens. We're not supposed to be living there but we're homeless again. My mom has to do a storage run and I enjoy long car rides, so I join her. I have to get my textbooks for school. It's the only thing I've ever had any control over—grades. School was my paradise away from home where I can blend into the background. I've never had a lot of friends, but my teachers always liked me. My mom is having an episode. She's screaming and cursing in her made-up language that sounds like a mixture of German and gibberish. She wants me to put the textbooks into storage. I tell her I need them, and she tells me we'll come back. But my mother is unpredictable and not very reliable, so I put no trust in her words and cling to the books, my arms wrapped around their spines. My mother

becomes frustrated and gets in the car; I go to open my side and it's locked. I
yell for my mom to open the door, but she starts to drive. I run beside the car,
clawing at the door handle, but she's going too fast and I'm out of breath. I
watch the car peel off until it's no longer in sight, and start to cry. "How could
she leave me?" replays in my head as I start to walk down the highway. Tears
stream down my face. I don't know my way back to my grandma's, but I know
I can't stay at the storage facility. A Latinx lady pulls her car over and asks me
if I need help. I see the rosary beads wrapped around her rearview mirror
and nod yes. Me and my mom have hitchhiked with strangers several times
before, so I hop in her car. She's very kind and soft spoken, nothing like my
mother. She's asking me questions, but all I can give her is my grandmother's
address. We make it. I thank Jehovah for sending me one of his angels and
proceed to tell my grandmother what happened. She freaks out. Long story
short, my mother had a change of heart and went back for me, but I was gone
so she called the police. They ended up coming to my grandma's and taking
my mom to a mental hospital because she clearly was not taking her medication. She was there for a month. I missed my mother, but it was also a relief
to have a break from her.

I'm sixteen and homeless. Me and my mom had been living out of her
car and showering at the YMCA. It's autumn in New York and slightly chilly
outside. Me and my grandma got into an argument, and she called my high
school and told them I was homeless to spite me. They set me up at "A Friend's
House"—a short-term shelter for homeless or runaway youths. None of the
parents here care about their children. None of them try. My mom didn't try.
Two months later I was freed from my "youth support" prison and moved
into a basement studio apartment with my mom.

I'm twenty, visiting my mom at a different mental hospital. She's been
there for about two weeks. I give her a hug because I miss her so much. They
have her on really strong tranquilizers. Her cheeks are sunken in, and her
eyes glazed over. She gives me a weak smile and tells me she's happy to see
me. She's talking really slow. The medication is really strong. I smile and hold
back tears. It's extremely painful for me to see my mother in this state, in this
place, again. I sit with her for an hour as she struggles to keep her eyes open.
Before I leave, I stop at the bathroom, lock the door, and cry. Breathing heavy
through sobs. I don't know what to do or how to help her.

Fast Forward to the Pandemic

Poem 1: Everything was the same

I chuckled at the world as my everyday reality bled into the lives of the middle class. Food pantries have never been foreign to me. Government assistance lines where acquiring Section 8 felt like the lottery. Can I trade you some food stamps for money, because the products with the red label are sold out again. People are starving in the streets, sleeping on the concrete but this has never been foreign so why should I worry about you when you never cared about me? Welcome to my cookie cutter piece of poverty, I hope you enjoy your stay here, until the government sets you free. Until life returns to normal and the memories of your misfortune are a bad dream. Me and the rest of the forgotten will be waiting for the people to pull back the curtain exposing the rotted roots of our societal tree.

Poem 2

Quality Time
& that was our thing
Whether it be
Jumbos
New York
Fortune
Saffron
Golden Corral
Buffet
We always went
To buffets
& we always
Had 2 plates
Plus dessert
& that was our thing

Watching
Netflix
Hulu
Cable
Movies
Shows
Except for
Horror
That was our thing

I hadn't seen my mom in a month because I didn't want to spread any unwanted pathogens. Unfortunately, when you live in low-income housing, it can be hard to social distance. Check the mail, germs. Do the laundry, germs. Use the elevator, germs. With so many shared facilities, how is she supposed to stay safe? The virus will spread the same way the bed bugs did.

My mom calls me, coughing violently. She can barely speak. My heart drops because all I can think about are the thousands of people who have already lost their lives to the virus. If my mom died, no one would know. No one would notice. I'm the only person who cares. Unless my neighbors' noses give way to the smell of rotting flesh. I would be the one to find her body. I get off the phone and cry outside. The room I rent is tiny and I don't want people to hear me. I ask my friends for a favor, and they agree to drive me two hours north to my mother's apartment. She refuses to go to the doctor, so I come bearing gifts. Vitamin C pills, Tylenol, cough drops, oranges, vegetables, fruits, honey, lemon, ginger. I go straight to the kitchen and start making lentil soup. I will heal her from the inside. After a few days, when I monitor her temperature closely, her fever breaks. She has a bit of a lingering cough, but I think she's going to be okay.

Poem 3

Cold, wet down
My face
Past my cheek
To my lips
My eyes must

Be salty
And out of
Nowhere idk
Why I'm crying
I pressed my palms
Against my eye sockets
Until they were soaked
And my breathing
became depressed
I just want these feelings to
Melt away.

2 Weeks Later (April 24th): Moving Day

I'm back in Brooklyn for three days and all I can think is what am I doing here? My landlady is a kind woman who understands I currently have no income. Normally, I'm a waitress but restaurants are shut and getting through to unemployment has been difficult. I'm on a rent freeze but my mother needs me. What am I doing here? I tell her I'm moving; we hug and say our goodbyes. She will be missed. My friends and I proceed on the journey two hours north once more, but this time my life is piled in the trunk and backseat. I arrive at my destination. My mind is at ease, this is where I need to be.

The New Normal

January 2021

Happy New Year!

I woke up at 5 a.m. to use the bathroom and found my mother on the toilet. She looked like she was on her deathbed and told me she had been there all night. She couldn't stop peeing. I called a friend and we rushed her to a VA clinic. After some blood work they told me that my mother's sugar was over 600 and she had type 2 diabetes. I sat with my mask on in the waiting room all day until the doctor finally told me that they had to keep her overnight to stabilize her blood sugar. They told us she was lucky that she came in today because if we had waited any longer, she would have slipped into a diabetic coma.

My mother was on the same floor as COVID patients, but she was not allowed to be released unless someone could administer the insulin. She had a long-standing fear of needles, and she was too panicked to poke herself. I ended up rushing back to the hospital two days later to listen to a crash course on living with diabetes. I remembered enough to make do and was able to bring her home. I checked her blood; she winced. I put the needle in her belly; she winced. Every time I mess up, we have to try again, and I see the sadness in her face. I go to the bathroom and cry. All the things I do, and I still can't protect you.

May 2021

We're both finally vaccinated. My mom got Moderna last month and I got my final dose of Pfizer on the 10th. Being vaccinated has taken away so much anxiety for us and it feels like we're finally seeing the light at the end of the pandemic tunnel. I also now serve as my mom's personal nutritionist, reading labels and looking for sugar alternatives. Furthermore, she's become a pro at checking her blood sugar and giving herself insulin. We've gotten into a routine and we're both doing our part. The weather is getting warm, and vaccinations have opened for all adult age groups. I'm feeling hopeful.

Mental Illness During COVID-19

The problems of the pandemic have been amplified for people with mental illnesses. According to public health researchers, "having a severe mental illness during the COVID-19 pandemic can quickly become a death sentence. These groups often have lifestyles that increase their risk for contracting coronavirus and have other underlying health conditions that raise their risk for developing more serious cases of COVID-19 if they contract the virus. Mental health issues often coincide with a unique set of challenges that make it difficult for people to access even the most basic necessities, such as food, medications, stable housing, and health care."[1] Furthermore, Black communities have always been under-resourced for mental health access which has been intensified by the pandemic. As the American Psychiatric Association notes, "Only one-in-three African Americans who need mental health care receive it"; "African Americans often receive poorer quality of care and lack access to culturally competent care."[2] Further, as Darcel Rockett writes, "Those who come in complaining of symptoms of mood disorders are less likely to get that diagnosis when they walk out."[3] In addition, in the first phases of the pandemic, people of color contracted COVID-19 at higher rates than their white counterparts. The COVID Tracking Project explained in 2021: "Nationwide, Black people are dying at 2.5 times the rate of white people."[4] Black people are also at a higher risk of being homeless. The combination of all of these factors puts Black people with severe mental illness at a much higher risk for contracting and transmitting COVID-19.

Parting Words

People with mental illnesses are often cast away by society as broken or devalued. This is especially true for Black people who are on the lower end of the societal hierarchy. The government continues to fail my mother time and time again. There isn't much of a support system and the health care system often lacks compassion for people like her. During this time, many of my mother's physical and mental health doctors canceled appointments and still continue to cancel appointments. Since it's so easy for this group to slip through the cracks and become forgotten, a lot of pressure falls on me as well as other caretakers and family members to step up where society has not. At times it was very hard for me to provide stability for her or myself, however through personal research and trial and error I have managed to create a routine and sense of security in our lives. While I'm happy to help my mother in any way possible, not everyone who is in her situation has been fortunate enough to have someone in their corner. The less fortunate often end up homeless and die prematurely, which is unfair. The world refuses to look at the pain it's causing and take responsibility for the people it sacrifices. Society fails to realize that every person is one traumatic event away from becoming disabled mentally or physically. Disabled people are not some annoyance that will eventually disappear; they are human beings who deserve love and compassion. My hope is that one day everyone will see these people as I do.

The Advocate

Growing up
In the gutter
Gave me a bird's-eye view
Of inequality.
At the fault of society
Someone tell me
Where is our Justice?
As people like my mother
Sleep on the street
Lungs too tight to breathe
Hospitals at capacity
Somebody tell me
Where is our humanity?
Cast aside for a person
Who is more able bodied
My mother risked her life
For a country that continues
To tell her she's undeserving.
VA hospitals missing doctors
As the chaos unfolds
I hope you rejoice
In your comfort
Built from our bodies,
Blood, sweat & tears
After years of silence
When the world asks
My mother
"who loved you?"
I'll be there to say I did.

CHAPTER 7

From Ahuehuetitla to Brooklyn: Immigrant Life Under COVID-19

Raúl Vaquero

It's March 18, 2020, a Wednesday afternoon in Union Square. It will turn out to be my last day of work and soon enough it will be my last day of in-person classes for my last semester of college. It's a strange scene. Usually, this part of NYC is packed with office workers, students, and pedestrians bumping into each other, rushing to their daily commute. Today the streets are nearly empty; it seems like many people decided to stay home, at least those who have that type of luxury. There are people out here still working: charging, lifting, breaking, building, or driving, but no one really pays attention to those people. Not while the rich treat NYC like their playground.

Little do they realize many of those people are immigrants. In fact, about one in four workers in New York is an immigrant. Yet they generally lack access to federal aid programs such as Medicaid, food stamps, and Temporary Assistance for Needy Families. As the son of immigrant parents, I would know. My parents and relatives recount the injustices they face on an everyday basis, from subtle discrimination to being unjustly treated in the workplace. "*Si, no molesta, pero estamos aquí por el bien de ustedes*," they would often say. How selfless of them. How unfair it is to them, to my neighbor next door and down the hall and across the street and around the block. They all ought to be home, but that's not how things work in the United States of America.

In 1882 the US Congress established the public charge rule for the sake of allowing the government to deny a visa to anyone who, "is likely at any time to become a public charge"—but without defining what "public charge" means.

Under the Trump administration, the "public charge rule" was interpreted broadly to reduce the number of people who were eligible for green cards and other visas, by penalizing those on any form of government assistance.[1] The Trump administration defined a public charge as an "alien" who receives one or more public benefits. This rule unabashedly targeted poorer immigrants using a "'merit-based'" system grounded in racist ideologies. Over the years the rule has been subjectively enforced. For example, in the early twentieth century, immigration officials on Ellis Island used the law to bar immigrants who were "likely to become public charges as an effective means of denying entry to Jewish immigrants."[2] The Trump administration used this rule to incite hatred, fear, and long-lasting trauma, a potent reminder that there is no safety net for immigrants to ward off sickness or hunger. My family and community faced the brunt of that.

It's March 19. Every Thursday I visit my parents. The neighborhood I moved to gives off the same calm vibe it does every day, unlike Flatbush, my parents' block, which is always loud and vibrant. Today things were quiet. Not a soul on the stoops or police sirens declaring ownership of the neighborhood. I can't imagine Tony, my now-deceased neighbor, seeing such a spectacle. With a big cigar on the side of mouth, he would tell us stories about what went down in Flatbush during the 1970s and '80s. Ever since the white flight of the 1980s, cops in the neighborhood have been an everyday thing. He says the blackout of '77 and former mayor Giuliani amped up the presence of the police. So with this eerie quiet, I knew today would be the last day I came to visit them for a while. My mom wasn't looking too good. I hope it's just a fever. News about my dad's only brother being in the hospital filled me with doubt. *Virgencita* please watch over her.

It's Tuesday evening, March 24. I got the news from my little sister that "*papa y mama se lo pasan tirados en la cama.*" This is news I thought I'd never hear. They wouldn't allow it—my dad can't go a day without working, and my mom can't go a minute without doing something. She often tells us that she'll get all the rest she needs when it's time for her to go. I'm not ready for that. I turn on the television for the sake of distracting myself, but the headlines about the virus only stress me out even more: "20-Somethings Now Realizing That They Can Get Coronavirus, Too"; "*Gobernador de Nueva York pide 30,000 ventiladores para los afectados por coronavirus*"; "Density Is New York City's Big 'Enemy' in the Coronavirus Fight."

My mind spins: Did my dad catch it from his workplace or did my mom catch it while running errands? Who else might be sick? I call my aunt who lives upstairs from my parents. She picks up and before she even says a word, she's coughing her lungs out. My parents were like that just a few days ago. She mentions to me that uncle wasn't feeling too well either and thinks he might have passed it on to her. What does this mean for my younger cousins? With school out, what are they going to eat or learn? Before another thought even crosses my mind, my cousin calls me. His dad, my father's only brother, is on a ventilator. He's tested positive and they think he might not make it. I think back to what *el Vicegobernador de Tejas* said: "*Los abuelos están dispuestos a morir por coronavirus para no dañar la economía.*" Who in their right mind would say such a thing? That forcibly frames the loss of the elderly as an equal exchange for sustaining the economy. He might be undocumented and old, but who died and appointed you the spokesperson for someone else's life?

It's March 25. I got word from my siblings that our parents aren't okay and that my *tio* from upstairs is too sick to get out of bed. How are my cousins, Christian and Danny, going to survive? They're only ten and seven years old. It's a forty-minute walk from my place to theirs. I have to do it, because how else are they going to eat if my aunt and uncle are coughing their lungs out like my parents? I get a blocked caller ID number calling me. "Raúl, I'm scared. Are my parents going to be okay?" I realized shortly after that it's Christian. I didn't know what to say. All I could do was share the little positivity I had left. "They'll be okay, I'll be dropping off some food soon, I made all your favorites," I say in an effort to cheer them up. I hear Danny crying in the background. Can she hear through my lies or is she just as scared as I am? Christian explains to me that "Danny is scared that someone is going to come while our mom and dad are sick." I know exactly who that someone is. She's imagining that ICE will take advantage of her parents while they're bedridden, come to the house, and take them away. "Danny, it's going to be okay, no one is going to come. Everyone has been ordered to stay home and that means even those bad people." Is this one of those times when it's okay to lie? This sucks. Things are only going to get worse, and I don't want to lose anybody.

It's April 16, my younger sister's birthday. Three weeks in and their road to full recovery is slow. Not just for them, but for all my *tios, tias,* and *vecinos.* In total, twenty-seven neighbors and relatives tested positive. The times then were extremely uncertain and far too riddled with anxiety to do anything other than pray, prepare, and juggle coursework for the sake of securing a degree they would be proud of. A degree that echoes the voices of my parents chanting *"si se puede"* or *"si trabajas duro y con ganas se puede lograr lo que sea en este país."* Despite them having experienced blatant racism, they continue to buy into this American dream that fails to take into account that we live under an umbrella of racial capitalism and white supremacy. This is evident as my little brother informs me that Dad's cell phone continues to ring on hourly intervals—as if it weren't clear the first time he picked up that he was too sick to come into work. Luckily, my father has a union that protects his absence. He's the only one who does. My uncles promptly returned to work as soon the body aches and coughs became more bearable. According to one uncle, the store owner wasn't even wearing a mask when he arrived, despite knowing that he was still positive. This man was completely disconnected from reality. All that mattered to him was business and his money.

It's April 27, and the Flatbush area continues to remain in a red COVID rating. This means an area reported COVID-19 test positivity rates higher than 10%, while other wealthier, whiter neighborhoods like Park Slope and the Upper West Side made it out quick, first yellow (experiencing less than 3% of positivity tests) and are now green. Absolutely clear of COVID-19. You would think this kind of discrepancy is new, but as historian Kathryn Olivarius argues in "The Dangerous History of Immunoprivilege," it has a long and sordid history.[3] In the Deep South in the nineteenth century, the threat of yellow fever

> was wielded as a weapon. . . . Pro-slavery theorists used yellow fever to argue that racial slavery was natural, even humanitarian, because it allowed whites to socially distance themselves; they could stay at home, in relative safety, if black people were forced to labor and trade on their behalf. . . . High mortality, it turns out, was economically profitable for New Orleans's most powerful citizens because yellow fever kept wage workers insecure, and so unable to bargain effectively. . . . The burden was on the working classes to get acclimated, not on the rich and powerful to invest in safety net infrastructure.[4]

It's September 8th, and this current reality of ripping parents and children from each other at the US border has given rise to unfathomable trauma. The Trump administration has gone above and beyond to systematically pursue a policy of family separation. Using this system historically designed to scare people from coming when they're fleeing desperate circumstances with no alternative is inhumane. This is an American tragedy with a long history and a cynical euphemism—the media naming it "family separation." These families aren't being separated, they are being ripped apart, torn apart, and it needs to be called what it is. By definition, this is torture. This is government-sanctioned child abuse, and this is on the Trump administration.

It's September 16th and at the current moment there are an estimated 5,400 immigrant children and parents and counting who are in the hands of the US government.[5] This ruthless harm is promoted by policymakers and government officials who are systematically tearing families apart and not held accountable, despite the fact that President Trump signed an executive order supposedly ending the policy of child separation in 2018.[6] The ACLU alleges that there have been more than one thousand family separations since that executive order.[7] More recently *Pro Publica* reported on how the Trump administration has used the coronavirus as a pretext to circumvent the normal legal protections allowed to migrant children.[8] Since March, ICE has circulated thousands of migrant children through hotel black sites,[9] making it virtually impossible for lawyers and advocates to locate them.[10] Instead, they're being deported en masse to "prevent the introduction of COVID-19 into the US"[11]—even though many of the deported children have tested negative. This is a complete shit show.

But the stage for these policies was set way before Trump even entered the White House. In 1994, the Clinton administration put into place a policy called "prevention through deterrence"—which continued through both Democratic and Republican administrations.[12] This led to an expanded wave of border infrastructure--with the idea that it would force migrants to undergo an even more dangerous and deadlier journey and thus act as a deterrent. The Bush administration followed by creating DHSA and expanded the border patrol exponentially.[13] Then came Obama who deported more people than any other president in all of US history.[14] To this day his words continue to ring loudly: "No matter how decent they are, no matter their reasons, the 11 million who broke these laws should be held accountable."[15] The audacity, the hypocrisy, the betrayal, the dangers of representational politics.

This idea that it used to be easier to cross the border runs counter to the stories of my uncle who arrived during Truman's presidency through the bracero program, but quickly returned home after experiencing severe and unjust exploitation. Through his work as a cotton picker and later as a machine operator preparing the fields, he would retell the story to my father and their younger siblings of how they were stripped of their clothes to be fumigated at the processing center, which irritated his entire body and much later in life caused him to lose a leg. He told it to them with a sense of humor to mask this dark past. Despite not being alive to hear these stories, the current iteration of this mess hits me personally.

Fast forward and it's June 2022 and President Joe Biden is in office. He's used executive action to unravel some of the Trump administration's bureaucratic rulings. Biden's first target was the "public charge" rule, which to no surprise was met with pushback from fourteen Republican state attorneys who claim that Biden was bypassing rules around making new federal regulations. Despite this rebuff, the Department of Homeland Security (DHS) released a notice of proposed rulemaking and called for comment by April 25th.[16] This attempt to invite the general public to chime in on affairs that will ultimately impact those who are excluded from leaving any commentary is concerning.

But despite doing away with some of the most glaring things, Biden has largely continued the bipartisan pattern of the past century of treating immigrants like essential labor with unessential lives—to the point that Texan Republican county judges and sheriffs for the last several years have equated immigrants with an invasion, a war, with people invading communities and causing crime. If there's any crime being committed it is the crime of seeking safety. Yet the weaponization of fear creates policies that allow deportations to continue through the contentious utilization of Title 42, a policy implemented during the COVID-19 pandemic, enabling the expulsion of migrants at the border without due process. In the blink of an eye, the opportunity of finding safety is taken away. Mouths are left gaping; all attention is at the border. All while the immigration court system continues to remain too ill-equipped to help those who have been here for years investing thousands of dollars in lawyers, applications, and time with pending cases. They are forced to remain in limbo for months and most often years, waiting for some kind of resolution. Waiting for some kind of work permit. Waiting for the opportunity to create roots, for the opportunity to be treated like the productive members of society they are. However, the reality is the system of immigration in this country is broken and has been broken for a long time. There are millions of migrant workers here working, who kept working through the pandemic with no existing health care or sick days, waiting to no longer be treated like faceless immigrants.

On a personal note, I'm back at Union Square but now as a teacher. I graduated from Brooklyn College, completed a master's degree at Bank Street

College of Education, and started working full-time as an English teacher
and immigrant liaison at the International High School of Union Square,
teaching ninth and tenth graders. It's a special place and my family is proud.
However, we continue to deal with the aftermath of COVID-19, which has
had lasting health implications, including respiratory issues for my parents.
During Trump's presidency, my aunt and uncle were discouraged by their
lawyer from seeking governmental assistance due to the public charge rule.
Struggling to make ends meet was nothing new, just another day.

Despite these challenges, I find fulfillment in serving the socio-emotional
and academic needs of the representatives of America's future, the recently
immigrated youth. Because of the pandemic and global economic fallout, this
year's student demographic hails largely from Ambato, Ecuador, who mentioned that tiendas on end were already on the verge of closing. Once the pandemic hit, *todo se acabo*. This, along with other unknown external factors,
forced families to send their kids on their own. Personal narrative assignments
revealed their strenuous journey to the United States. Some would lament having to relive the journey they had barely survived but persisted in telling their
tale of gratitude, injustice, perseverance, and cruelty. Some were fortunate
enough to arrive in NYC by plane, while others recounted their experiences
crossing by car, bus, and or train though Colombia, Nicaragua, Guatemala,
and Mexico before even arriving in the United States. A few students deeply
inhale and exhale, gazing outside the ninth-floor window, as they vividly detail
their days in detention centers, emphasizing the profound trauma they have
endured. Unfortunately, their suffering does not end there.

In October 2022, Mayor Adams declares a state of emergency as governors play politics and bus migrants to New York—to teach New Yorkers a
lesson—and Manhattan hotels become a refuge for thousands. This year's
student demographic is a kaleidoscope—countries that were already in a precarious state when the global fallout of the pandemic further exacerbated the
hardships faced by their citizens. Unlike the previous year, where the majority
of students came from one specific area, this year students hail from different
parts of South and Central America as well as Africa, the Middle East, South
Asia, and Southeast Asia, carrying stories of having survived unspeakable
conditions, including hunger and homelessness. The dire economic circumstances they face here in NYC are inseparable from the collapse of their home
country. As the school year progresses many families of students mentioned
difficulty finding employment and adjusting to the fast-paced, inequitable

demands of the city. A few families decided not to return and instead relocated to other states like Connecticut, New Jersey, Florida, Minnesota, Texas, or Pennsylvania. Other families mentioned struggling profusely but refrained from relying on government assistance, considering it rude and a reflection of poor character. However, they grapple with the harsh reality that not seeking help entails working long hours for insufficient pay. This unspoken shame associated with accepting aid implies a failure to cope. A failure to make it *en la gran manzana*. All because this concept of receiving, accepting, and begging for supplemental assistance is considered a burden. The burden of this belief, intensified by the public charge rule, is rooted in a long-standing history and warrants a re-evaluation. Fundamental health care should be a basic right not dependent on charity.

The public charge rule continues to be the metaphor for immigrant life in this country. As the pandemic laid bare, this country wants our work, celebrates it, and would not function without it. But our lives, our health and well-being, and our family's health and safety, they make clear, are *not* their responsibility.

CHAPTER 8

COVID-19 Deportations

Anthony Salazar Vazquez

January 29, 2020

The unimaginable happened. ICE agents took my uncle at 5 a.m. this past Sunday. They banged on the door, yelling to open up. You could even hear some officers walking in our backyard. It felt like a raid. I was afraid that they would take my mom and dad. What would happen if they did? How would I survive on my own? What about my school? Would I need to leave school and start working full-time to support myself?

My uncle has been living in this country for twenty-five years with my family and has never committed a crime. It's unfair! I hope he is allowed to stay and continue living with us. I worry about our finances. New York City is very expensive, and my uncle helps pay the bills.

February 7, 2020

My uncle's Master Calendar Hearing is on Monday, and we still haven't found an attorney for him. My sister, Catherine, has reached out to several organizations for pro bono representation. I have gone to see private attorneys and they tell me that the best option for my uncle is to ask for a voluntary departure because there is no law that would allow him to stay. The attorney explained to us that voluntary departure is when a person agrees to leave the country through their own means. We can buy my uncle his ticket to leave and make sure he lands in the closest airport to the small town in Mexico that our family is from, and he would not be barred from legally returning to the United States in the future.

Catherine went to go see my uncle at Bergen County Jail, where he is detained. She tells me that he is his usual self, telling jokes and laughing as if he weren't locked up but that it was a shock seeing him in an orange jumpsuit. He calls often throughout the day and Mom talks to him over the phone.

February 19, 2020

I went with Catherine to visit my uncle today. Walking through those cold hallways made me wonder how he was doing. It was shocking to see him through glass and have to talk to him over a phone. It was as if he were a dangerous criminal. He didn't look much different and his hopeful and joyful character hadn't changed. He told me new jokes he had learned from his cell-mates, he was laughing and smiling, and he kept talking with me as if a piece of glass wasn't separating us. He and Catherine talked about the past-due bills he left, and she gave him the news that she has an attorney for him. I know she is stressed about that.

There's talk about a virus called COVID-19 that was first found in China spreading around the world. A case was already confirmed in the United States, but nothing in New York. Probably just another swine flu. It'll pass.

March 3, 2020

A lot has happened since the last time I wrote. The first case of COVID-19 was confirmed in New York. Everything is starting to shut down. We aren't allowing guests in our house, and we wash our hands before doing anything.

We're telling my uncle to stay safe and wash his hands often.

March 8, 2020

COVID is spreading quickly and we're afraid. We started wearing gloves and masks when leaving the house. Whenever we come inside, we must throw the gloves and mask away. Mom is a vulnerable person because she has type 2 diabetes.

My uncle tells me that he kind of likes being detained. He says that he has nothing to worry about. He spends his time watching TV, playing chess, and he doesn't have to work to be able to pay bills. But is that worth being locked up? I think he is trying to be strong for us. He looks like he's losing weight, and he tells me that he does not like the food they serve. Catherine told him that she isn't going to visit anymore because of COVID. Traveling to him is too risky.

I underestimated this thing.

March 13, 2020

Everything is different. Businesses are closing, and more and more people are starting to wear masks. We don't go out anymore. Dad told his boss that he will be working fewer days so he doesn't expose himself too much. I don't know if that is a good idea. Our family depends on his income, and if he works less, we might need to make budget cuts. Well, everything is closing, so we won't be able to spend money on unnecessary things, so maybe we can survive.

March 16, 2020

The office manager of the law office where I have worked the past five years called to say that we have to apply for unemployment, but he promised that I can go back to work once the office is allowed to open again. We can barely find disinfecting wipes and hand sanitizer in stores and the ones we do find are crazy expensive.

My uncle only calls once a day now because, in an effort to prevent any virus spread, Bergen County is limiting the free time the inmates have. The news says that jails are a ticking bomb. If one person gets COVID, everyone there will!

My uncle has asthma and if he gets COVID, he might die. His attorney is helping him to get him released on a bond because he's at high risk.

March 23, 2020

I spoke with my uncle today. He and the other detainees are in their cells all day and are only allowed outside for thirty minutes. In that time he has to do everything: shower, get snacks, pick up his mail, and call us. Mom told him to only call to let us know he's okay. No long conversations with him anymore.

April 6, 2020

Everything is closed. The hospitals are overflowing with patients. Positive cases, death rates, and unemployment keep rising. Hospital beds and the number of ventilators keep decreasing. COVID is messing up the world. All we see on the news are images of hospitals, the coolers hospitals use to store the dead bodies, and the charts of how the numbers of infections rise.

I haven't even seen the outside world in weeks! I'm desperate to see friends and hang out. We keep FaceTiming to check in on each other.

Today is Mom's birthday. Catherine bought a small cake just for us. She says that although we're living in a very difficult time, we should still have some type of joy in our life.

April 12, 2020

My uncle tells me that he's still only allowed out of his cell for thirty minutes per day and that the TV is on all the time. He told me he hears the virus is really bad outside, but the ICE agents don't wear masks.

April 18, 2020

Today we did some grocery shopping. I was excited about going out, but scared about getting infected. We had to wait in a line outside to avoid over-crowding inside.

The most important thing is that I went outside for the first time in over a month. What a relief!

May 25, 2020

There's talk about a reopening soon. We are slowly flattening the curve. Hopefully, everything will go back to normal.

My uncle is finally allowed more time to go out. I think we're going to reach normality soon, something that seemed to be a dream. We're still awaiting trial for him.

June 18, 2020

The judge denied my uncle bail even when the attorney proved that my uncle is at risk because of his asthma. He was granted a voluntary departure and now we have to look for flights to take him to Mexico City. His hometown is a ten-hour bus ride from there.

June 22, 2020

My uncle's attorney told us that ICE is not allowing my uncle to leave on a commercial flight due to the risk of COVID. If only they considered that in his bail hearing! So ICE will follow a deportation process for my uncle. They will fly him to a town along the border, make him cross a bridge to Mexico, and abandon him and the other deportees on the other side.

According to his attorney, my uncle will be taken to Laredo, Texas, on July 7th. Catherine and I decided that I will travel to Laredo and cross over to Mexico, because of my Mexican citizenship. I will look for my uncle and we'll go to a hotel. On the next day, we will fly to Mexico City to meet Catherine and take him home.

We decide to do this because border towns in Mexico are some of the most dangerous places in Mexico. Often deportees get assaulted by criminals.

Aside from that, many people get lost in these towns because these are places they've never been before, and they don't know anyone. My uncle doesn't have a phone or much money to be able to get help, and even if he looks for help, he could get scammed. My family and I worry about what could happen to him.

July 6, 2020

Tomorrow I leave for Laredo, and I'm afraid of getting COVID. I'm going to wear a KN-95 mask, face shield, and gloves. I have bottles of travel-size hand sanitizer and disinfecting wipes.

Last week I went to the ICE offices to drop off a bag for my uncle. We packed him a T-shirt, pants, sneakers, socks, $50, KN-95 masks, and a burner phone with our numbers saved.

July 8, 2020

I made a stop in Houston before landing in Laredo. When I landed in Houston, I got a call from my uncle. ICE sent him across the border! I made sure the hotel allowed him to arrive a day earlier than we had planned.

I was supposed to cross to Mexico today, but I wasn't allowed because I don't have a Mexican passport. The border is closed for all nonessential travel. I'm going to have to fly tomorrow to Dallas, then Phoenix, then Hermosillo, and finally to Mexico City where I will meet up with Catherine. My uncle will be in Nuevo Laredo until his flight to Mexico City on Friday.

In Mexico City we will get a rental car so as not to use public transportation. When we pick up my uncle at the airport, we'll leave for his hometown and then drive back to the airport on Saturday, because our flight back to New York is on Sunday.

July 12, 2020

The past few days we've been traveling through Mexico nonstop. Right now, we're waiting to board the flight back home. I'm exhausted and my body is all sore. Once I get on that flight I'm going to sleep.

After months of not seeing my uncle, finally seeing him was a very special moment. He started talking about his other inmates and how each inmate had their own hidden talent. One inmate knew how to make bracelets out of worn-out T-shirts. Another one knew how to draw sketches and, as he told us, he pulled out some of the pieces that the detainee drew.

July 13, 2020

I slept the entire flight home (I didn't even notice when we took off or landed!). After landing, I went to take the COVID test. I have to wait ten to fourteen days for my results. The doctor told me to stay home for two weeks. Hoping for good results.

Today I woke up with a fever. Mom put me into quarantine so I'm in my room. I feel worse than before.

July 15, 2020

Fever check: over 100 degrees. Catherine is sick too, 102 degrees. Catherine, Mom, and Dad went to get tested for COVID too. Dad is having chest pains and trouble breathing. Mom is having fevers and body aches. I still haven't gotten my results. I hope it isn't COVID.

That's all. I'm too sick to write.

July 20, 2020

Catherine and I feel better. The house is a disaster. We have plastic taped everywhere and no one is allowed to be in the same room. If we want to leave our rooms, we have to wear our masks and gloves.

Mom and Dad got their COVID results already. They're positive. I still haven't gotten mine but, for sure I'll be positive. I was the first one to feel sick. My aunt is doing our grocery shopping. She leaves everything at our front door.

Dad has pneumonia and I've told him to go to the hospital because that could be deadly. He tells us he doesn't want to die alone and that he'd rather die at home. Catherine is in charge of Mom and Dad's medical care. She gives them their medicine and checks their temperature. I cook. We'll make it through.

July 28, 2020

I got my COVID results yesterday. Positive. I haven't had a fever for the past eight days. No body aches and no drowsiness. I went to get retested today.

Back in Mexico, no one is sick, but out of precaution they're in quarantine too.

August 2, 2020

Mom and Dad are feeling better. They went to get retested, and Mom came back negative. Dad is still positive. Now he's the only one in quarantine and not allowed to go out. Catherine and I are waiting for our results.

August 16, 2020

Catherine and I got our results back—negative. Finally, once again, I get to go out.

We're just waiting for Dad to test negative. He went a few days ago and we're expecting a result tomorrow.

My uncle and my relatives in Mexico didn't show any symptoms and tested negative for COVID.

August 17, 2020

Good news! We're all negative!

This time that we were sick taught me a lot. To really appreciate life and those around us. I've never felt this sick before. If it wasn't for them deporting my uncle, I would never have needed to fly—I would never have gotten COVID.

End Note

When the COVID-19 pandemic abruptly arrived in the United States, the nation's stagnant and careless response caused the rapid spread of the virus throughout every city and town. While many people emphasized the drastic impacts the pandemic had on working-class communities, essential workers, and the unemployed, we seem to forget, or choose not to talk about, the inmates in ICE detention centers.

In 2020, ICE detained 19,068 people.[1] Many detainees released during the pandemic have described the horrors they experienced in the detention centers. ICE kept the inmates in overcrowded and unsanitary conditions and did not even test the inmates.[2] These conditions made ICE detention centers a ticking time bomb for a rapid, and even deadly, COVID-19 spread. ICE distributed masks to detainees late, failed to report infections, pressured staff and guards to work regardless of their health, refused to enforce mask wearing among their agents, and denied the release of high-risk people.[3]

Not only were living conditions not safe in the detention centers, but ICE also continued to transfer inmates between centers during the pandemic. And COVID-19 spread. In early May 2020, the first COVID-19-related death of an ICE detention center inmate was reported. His name was Carlos Escobar-Mejia, a fifty-seven-year-old Salvadoran man. Weeks before Escobar-Mejia's death, on April 21, four detainees from Butler County Jail were transferred to the detention center where Escobar-Mejia was being kept.[4] On April 13, The Butler County sheriff's office reported the first confirmed case of COVID-19 in Butler County Jail.[5]

ICE also continued to deport people. From January to August 2020, ICE sent roughly 450 deportation flights to fifteen different countries in Latin America and the Caribbean. Eleven of the fifteen countries reported that deportees arrived with COVID-19.[6] These deportations contributed to the global spread of the virus, especially to a region that lacks the necessary resources to fight the pandemic. At one point, 20% of the total number of known COVID-19 cases in Guatemala were people deported from the United States.[7] ICE's exportation of COVID-19 was so severe that the Honduran Ministry of Health required all deportees to be tested for COVID-19 upon arrival. Many of the deportees that tested negative later developed symptoms and tested positive.[8]

Just like the federal government response, ICE's management of their detention centers during the pandemic was irresponsible, horrific, and inhumane. "By August 1, almost 5.5 percent of total US [confirmed COVID-19] cases . . . were attributed to spread from ICE detention centers."[9] ICE transported COVID-19 on a national and international scale, worsening the situation. Between May and August 2020, over 245,000 COVID-19 cases emerged from ICE's detention centers. If ICE were its own country, it would have ranked sixteenth in the global case rate.[10]

Just like my uncle, many people's lives were put at risk because of ICE. My uncle was one of the fortunate few who did not get infected with COVID and made it to their home countries healthy. In the correction facility where my uncle was staying, the officers did not follow the safety protocols of wearing their masks inside and left the detainees in a single cell without enough room to be physically distanced from one another. My uncle's story is just a single person's experience, yet there are many people who do not get the chance to tell their story because they are alone in this country or are in their native countries trying to move forward with their lives, or, for far too many, because they didn't live to tell their story at all.

CHAPTER 9

Chinatown Through a Pandemic:
A Phoenix Rising

Kayla Gutierrez

My grandmother didn't leave her house for five months.

This is not an exaggeration. She did not set foot outside of her house once from March 2020, when New York City went into quarantine, until August 23rd, five months later. Not even for groceries or to go to a laundromat. This was because she feared for her life. How could she not, given the state of the world at the time? But unlike others who feared the deadly virus making waves globally, she was afraid of simply existing. As COVID-19 wreaked havoc on everyone's lives, more and more individuals expressed their anger and irritation at the death of their old normal. Unfortunately, this often came at the expense of safety for individuals who possessed features associated with an East Asian background.

Let's backtrack a bit to February 2020, when my mother, a Chinese-American, was being offered a managerial position at the medical office where she worked. She had over thirty years of experience and was already managing the rest of her coworkers, just without the title and the pay associated with it. Eventually, my mom was recognized for her hard work and was offered that managerial position. Yet only three weeks later, my mom was fired. The office explained that due to COVID-19 regulations requiring them to minimize occupancy, there was a lack of patients, and thus a lack of income. Because of this, my mom's former boss explained, people would have to be let go. Although she was not the only Asian American working there at the time, she was the only person with East Asian features and the only person in the office who lost her job.

To be honest, it wasn't really a surprise that my mom was fired. She worked at the front desk of a medical facility greeting patients during a pandemic that East Asians became the face of—when even the most visible politician at the time, President Trump, labeled COVID the "China Virus" or the "Kung Flu."[1] COVID was not just "Chinese made"; Asians themselves were seen *as* the virus. And for many Asian Americans, losing their job was no longer a question of if, but rather when.[2] As time passed and COVID spread its damage, unemployment rates among Asian Americans skyrocketed: "In February 2020, Asian Americans in New York City had a jobless rate of 3.4%—however, Asian American unemployment soared to 25.6% by May 2020, the largest increase among all major racial groups."[3] Hate and discrimination began to rise and be reported. In March 2020, the Stop Asian American and Pacific Islander hate website received 2,373 anonymous reports of hate and discrimination.[4]

If you take a walk through Manhattan's Chinatown, you can see how different it is from Tribeca or Midtown. There are no picture windows or clean, tall buildings with doormen. The buildings in Chinatown hold different stories of success: stories of immigrants living in tenements, creating a community, surviving discrimination, and working in factories, restaurants, and fish markets, trying to ride the American Dream. You would see hard work and unity, everyone supporting each other, donating during Lunar New Year, and doing group Tai Chi in the morning. My family has lived in Chinatown since the 1970s; both my mother and I grew up there and still live there today. When I was young, the children of the neighborhood frequently met up to play, so everyone felt connected, and this is still the case now. To me and my mother, Chinatown has always felt like a very close community. Although people had their differences, and the melting pot of different Asian cultures often led to some divisions, this sense of connection and mutual understanding was widespread in Chinatown. There was never a day it wasn't crowded. Even in the rain and snow, tourists and locals mingled.

Under COVID, everything changed. People isolated themselves, and walking the empty streets felt somewhat shameful. You never knew if someone was going to be violent toward you, so being away from others meant being safe. Seeing all the shuttered businesses and lack of street culture, it felt almost like I didn't belong here anymore. I am of mixed Dominican and Chinese heritage, and I often felt that I got weird looks, or people would stay away, or stores would try to sell me things at a tourist price because I didn't look "Asian" enough (and therefore must not be a Chinatown resident). "Storefront for rent" signs littered the streets, and entire blocks became lined with metal gates signaling the end of an era. And unfortunately, most of these places were restaurants I grew up eating in or stores I frequented. The ripped-out interiors of the buildings were the only reminders of past birthdays, banquets, and other celebrations. Chinatown was no longer Chinatown, known for being festive and a melting pot of cultures. It became more of a ghost town, losing much of the magic it had before.

Even before COVID-19 precautions were put in place nationwide, many Asian businesses experienced a decline in customer visits and sales, due to fears associated with the specific population. A UCLA study found that sales declined in Chinatown by more than three quarters starting from late January 2020, a time of year when the neighborhood is usually bustling due to Lunar New Year celebrations.[5] And unfortunately, many of these businesses lacked support from the government: businesses in Chinatown zip codes 10013 and 10038 were unable to get Small Business Services loans because the median area income was too high to be eligible for the program.[6] This was largely because these zip codes encompassed parts of Soho and Tribeca, two of Manhattan's wealthiest neighborhoods, which raised income averages above the eligibility level for the program. As a result, financial help from the government was trivial—only five thousand dollars to businesses that make less than fifty thousand per year and ten thousand to businesses that made one hundred thousand per year.[7]

It seemed like while the rest of the world slowly began to adjust to living under COVID, the Asian American community was thrust even further into exile. Politicians stayed quiet about much hate Asians faced, due to fears of losing face or votes. Former President Trump created an environment in which anti-Asian racism and bullying seemed acceptable. So when New York City mayor Bill de Blasio announced his visit to Chinatown in April, to hear us out and bring awareness, we rejoiced. Finally, a step forward. A beacon of hope for Chinatown, for our culture, for our elderly. But just like the famous idiom predicted, we took two steps back.

From live broadcasting, I watched an interview with Mayor de Blasio and Patrick Mock, the manager of a small bakery at 46 Mott Street, in which Mock expressed the fear and pain that so many Chinatown residents felt during this difficult and scary time. He also said what he thought would help boost

Chinatown's visits and help keep many businesses, and people for that matter, alive. Mock's vision included closing Mott Street for restaurants and stores to use the space, and turning it into a night market, as well as starting a fund to make Chinatown more aesthetically pleasing to boost visits. But Mayor de Blasio turned his back and walked away, literally, just as Mock was expressing the need for help. De Blasio didn't even let Mock finish before stating that our struggles were "unfortunate" and preparing to leave.[8] The mayor stated that he cared about the city's people, but then did almost nothing for Chinatown. Despite Mock's plea for aid, Mott Street was not closed, and the businesses of Chinatown continued to see a decline.

To help keep Chinatown alive, many citizens and activists donated to Asian businesses. Welcome to Chinatown, a community organization and blog originally created many years ago to increase tourism and community within Chinatown, launched the Longevity Fund, which garnered $278,487 in donations to help fund Chinatown businesses. Forty small businesses in Chinatown were given $5,000 to help keep them afloat, and the rest of the funding was divided among elderly residents of Chinatown.[9] The nonprofit organization Chinatown Partnership also assisted small businesses by helping fund and construct outdoor eating establishments for Asian restaurants.[10] Their goal was to try to improve sales and foot traffic within Chinatown. Although these organizations strove to keep Chinatown afloat, neighborhood businesses still struggled.

If the mayor of the city you live in turns his back on the very people he swore to always have in mind, then who is going to help? It was another example of the Chinatown community being alone and unsupported. It also showed those hurting the community that they could get away with what they were doing. People continued to avoid Chinatown, except for those who came just to hurl abuse at the residents. Hate crimes against Asians began to rise, especially toward the elderly. A Pew Research article stated that "three-in-ten Asian adults (31%) say they have been subject to slurs or jokes because of their race or ethnicity since the outbreak [of COVID] began, compared with 21% of Black adults, 15% of Hispanic adults, and 8% of white adults."[11] Meanwhile, a different Pew Research article reported that a staggering 32% of Asian Americans feared being threatened or physically attacked—a higher percentage than any other ethnic or racial group during this time.[12]

The outrage at Mayor de Blasio's actions prompted a statement from the Mayor's Office: "New Yorkers are never afraid to share their thoughts, and we're grateful for [Mock's] ideas and advocacy for his community. We know COVID-19 has hit small businesses hard, and we're actively exploring more ways to help Chinatown recover."[13] One month later, Chirlane McCray, Mayor de Blasio's wife, announced a racial inclusion and equity task force, for Women, Black, and Latino businesses.[14] Yet businesses owned by Asian Americans, which were severely affected by racism on top of the pandemic, would not be included in the task force.[15]

The virus eased, but under the new normal, many Asian Americans continued to be afraid of being attacked by racist individuals blinded by hatred. And once again, the city failed the Asian American community, as abusers often got just a slap on the wrist before being let go. Consider the case of fifty-two-year-old Lee-Lee Chin-Yeung, who was pushed into a mailbox in Flushing Queens by Patrick Mateo.[16] Despite Yeung's daughter testifying to the racist statements Mateo made before the attack, the New York Police Department claimed to have found no basis for classifying the assault as a hate crime. Chin-Yeung was knocked unconscious and left with ten stitches. Then, hours later, Mateo was released from custody "under supervision." Although Mayor de Blasio spoke out against hate crimes toward Asian Americans, barely any action was taken by his administration to protect Asian Americans. The lack of government action has led to organizations such as SafeWalx, which relies on volunteers to walk elderly Asian Americans home safely, given the rise of anti-Asian hate crimes.[17]

Thinking about the hate my community receives makes my bones burn with rage. East Asians are being told we are the cause of a virus by many of the very same individuals who refuse to wear a mask and social distance, as if Asian Americans have not lost their loved ones, too. During a time of vulnerability, fear, and hardship, it feels as if the Asian American community is being left behind. Much of this has to do with the beliefs spread through the inaccurate "model minority" stereotype, as well as the failure of individuals in positions of power to protect us.[18] Asian Americans are severely underrepresented in leadership positions. A *New York Times* article found that Asians make up only 3% of political leadership positions within the United States, the lowest of any racial group.[19] Having so few Asian Americans in positions of civic power, coupled with public blame from the former president for the coronavirus, has created an openly discriminatory atmosphere.

Living in Chinatown during the pandemic was rough. With so little foot traffic, many establishments were forced to close; prices in the supermarket began to rise and locals bought things in bulk. The stock was also often sold out due to import delays and slowdowns in the United States as well as China. Being a person of mixed Asian/Latin descent during the pandemic presented challenges of its own. Looking at me, one might not initially be able to tell that I'm Asian. And my Hispanic last name often seals the deal for most that I am just Hispanic. Because of this, many of my Asian peers felt I was not at high risk for anti-Asian hate, and not at risk for any ostracization due to the virus because of my Asian ethnicity. These assumptions alienated me from my own community. On the other hand, many non-Asian individuals often felt comfortable being racist toward Asians in my presence because they didn't realize I am Asian or, in their opinion, I am not Asian *enough*, so I couldn't possibly care. I remember during the height of the pandemic I was having a text conversation with one of my peers who lived in Brooklyn. He told me he wouldn't be coming to Chinatown any time soon, followed by a bat, rat, and virus emoji. This was despite the fact that he lived in the part of Brooklyn that had the highest COVID-19 case rates at the time. But that wasn't the first time someone came to the conclusion that if you were Chinese, you had COVID or you were a super spreader. My grandma leaves her house now, though very rarely and not for long periods of time, to avoid any possibility of catching COVID or becoming a victim of hate.

So many of the hardships Asian Americans have faced during the pandemic stem from the labels imposed on us and the beliefs that are spread about who we are. The increase in anti-Asian hate and the lack of support from the government made us Asian Americans feel alone and afraid, forcing us to seek aid from each other to survive this pandemic. We struggled as a community and despite our needs being rejected and ignored, Chinatown has survived. Restaurants and businesses that have closed are now being replaced by new Asian establishments, and Chinatown has begun to slowly rebuild. In the face of systematic discrimination, we will be united and strong, never giving up fighting in the hopes that one day we will be treated equally.

CHAPTER 10

Black Lives Matter: COVID-19, Race, and Organized Abandonment

Rhea Rahman

On May 25, 2020, George Floyd was murdered by Minneapolis police officer Derek Chauvin. The nine-minute video of his execution circulated widely the next day on social media, prompting protests in Minneapolis and sparking a summer of national uprising unprecedented in scale. This spectacular display of the nation-state's disregard for Black life ignited public rage over the increasingly untenable conditions of white supremacy that were magnified by the pandemic, including: "the worst public health and economic crisis in generations, three and a half years of a divisive and chaotic presidential administration, a burgeoning white nationalist movement, and decades upon decades of growing economic inequality amid an increasingly threadbare social safety net."[1]

Despite not yet having any means to counter the virus, such as mass testing or vaccines, millions left the relative protection of their homes for the streets, deeming it safer to be outside protesting for a new world, than to continue to accept the status quo of the existing one. I had been watching demonstrations from the comfort of my parents' home in suburban Michigan. When at the beginning of the pandemic my mother asked me to come stay with her and my dad, though worried about my aging parents, I was reluctant. Yet after weeks of daily video calls from my mother, seeing the worry in her face as she could hear the constant sirens blaring from outside my windows in Brooklyn, I promised her that I would come home for the month of Ramadan. A few days after Eid, the uprising was just beginning. I was still in Michigan and anxious to get back to New York. When I saw a video on Twitter of an NYPD vehicle driving into a group of protestors in Brooklyn,[2] just blocks from my apartment, I resolved to return and join the people in the streets. My mother, who was staying up each night watching the protests on cable news, was terri-fied and wanted to postpone my return. "But my peonies are about to bloom," she pleaded, "just wait a few more days."

I didn't wait for the peonies. I rented a car and the next day I found myself ascending from the Holland tunnel to confront the largest police barricade I had ever seen. Between the number of in-street demonstrations and milita-rized police fortifications throughout downtown Manhattan, I feared that I wouldn't make it home to Brooklyn before the city's first official curfew since 1943.[3] The next day I was reunited with colleagues, comrades, and friends—meeting some in person for the first time—at a rally for racial justice in the NYC public education system. On a day with over twenty rallies, marches, and protests throughout the city,[4] we moved from one protest to another, avowing the movement's recognition that all forms of oppression are inter-connected. I felt part of a revolutionary call to invest in people over profits, as we dared to imagine a world in which Black Lives Matter and all the radical transformations our society would have to make for that to be possible.

While there were many catalysts for the uprising of 2020, the most signifi-cant groundwork was laid by the Black Lives Matter movement. Prompted by the murder of seventeen-year-old Trayvon Martin in 2012, BLM was initiated by three Black women organizers—Alicia Garza, Patrisse Cullors, and Opal Tometi. In 2013 when George Zimmerman was acquitted of Martin's mur-der, Garza posted the following on her social media account: *"Black people. I love you. I love us. Our lives matter, Black Lives Matter."* The last three words, Black Lives Matter, went viral and developed into a national, and then global, movement. BLM shifted national discourse by calling out systemic racism, white supremacy, and anti-blackness.[5] These terms and related grounded analysis have countered even the liberal "anti-racism" that views racism as an individual pathology and that ultimately upholds a system in which some lives are not as worthy of mattering as others.[6]

The statement itself—Black Lives Matter—defies the accepted disposability of Black life, the accepted invisibility of Black lives, the accepted hypervisibility of Black lives; it refuses the anti-Black normalization of slow death,[7] fast vio-lence,[8] and organized state abandonment.[9] And yet a movement to advocate for this most basic recognition of the humanity of Black lives spawned not only counter-movements and slogans such "All Lives Matter," but also prompted a number of political and popular efforts to label BLM a terrorist organization.[10] Both the power, and perceived threat, of Black Lives Matter is that to recognize anti-blackness as an implicit doctrine of the nation-state is to acknowledge the reality of white supremacy as normal, accepted, and status quo.

Just as BLM—and the uprising of 2020 as a particular moment in this movement—forces us to confront the taken-for-granted status quo that determines whose lives get to matter, so too do the powerful student pieces in this collection. Billie-Rae Johnson, Raúl Vaquero, Anthony Salazar Vazquez, and Kayla Gutierrez force a reckoning with what Ruth Wilson Gilmore has termed the state's "organized abandonment" of their loved ones.[11] Although the concept of state-organized abandonment refers to an apparent withdrawal of government support and programs, it names a *purposeful* strategy of the racial capitalist state to create and then exploit vulnerable communities. It names a racism that is not operationalized through an explicit intention to produce harm, but rather through the *willful* neglect of people, communities, and populations deemed surplus to the contemporary political economic order. Although the concept refers to a foundational logic in the governance of populations and environments, it is experienced materially and affectively at an individual level.[12] Portraying this material and affective experience is what these student autoethnographies do, and what makes them so powerful.

Having a mother who exists at multiple vectors of marginalization—Black, poor, a woman, and living with mental illness—Billie-Rae Johnson highlights a lifetime of her mother's life not mattering to anyone aside from herself. Describing in searing detail her mother moving in and out of assisted-living homes, living on and off the streets, without adequate care for her mental and physical health, Johnson impeccably spotlights the effects of organized state-abandonment: "Since it's so easy for this group to slip through the cracks and become forgotten about, a lot of pressure falls on me as well as other caretakers and family members to step up where society has not." And further, she denounces this abandonment as not by accident, but by design: "The world refuses to look at the pain it's causing and take responsibility for the people it sacrifices." And from the normalized, socially acceptable disregard for Billie-Rae Johnson's mother, Anthony Salazar Vazquez brings to light the institutionalized state-sponsored disposability of ICE detainees. When his uncle is detained and eventually deported by ICE, it is Salazar Vazquez and his sister who spend days traveling throughout Mexico to get their uncle to his home village safely, both contracting COVID-19 in the process. Whereas Kayla Gutierrez's Chinese grandmother did not leave her home for five months, Gutierrez foregrounds how in the absence of government support, members of the Chinatown community turn to each other to survive the manifold impacts of the pandemic. When Raúl Vaquero's parents, aunt, and uncle fall sick, Vaquero steps in to comfort his young nephew. Each narrative offers an example of confronting the state's organized abandonment with the tangible connections of family, care, and love. The students' writings are acts of care that make visible that which society has attempted (and failed) to render invisible. By placing into relief our collective apathy in the face of their loved ones' disposability, these students' acts of care incriminate us. Calling out our shared responsibility for the abandonment of their family members, we who encounter these words are called to act. Do we continue to ignore those we disregard, or do we respond and act otherwise?

Autoethnography and the Lived Experience of Racial Capitalism

Growing up
In the gutter
Gave me a bird's-eye view
Of inequality.

As Johnson conveys in the epigraph above, each piece reflects the situated position of the author, providing narratives that expose how dynamics such as racialization, gender, poverty, nationality, and mental health manifest and produce the social comorbidities exacerbated by the COVID-19 pandemic. As the uprising of 2020 amplified, it is the existing social fabric—the political economic order of racial capitalism—that renders some more vulnerable to illness and premature death. Autoethnography allows us to see in granular detail *how* institutional structures of white supremacy constitute social hierarchies, impacting individual lives and determining life choices. An inherently blurred genre operating at the intersections of the affective and the analytical, autoethnography brings forth the layered impacts of the pandemic on the most vulnerable.

For example, despite Black people dying of COVID at 2.5 times the rate of white people, even during the pandemic the virus was not the deadliest threat to Black lives.[13] Indicting a health care system that lacks compassion for people like her mother, Johnson's account highlights the ways Black communities are systematically under-resourced (and often go untreated) for mental and physical health. At the axis of multiple valences of racialized, state-rendered disposability, Johnson's mother is failed by the state and society, again and again. Beginning her piece with a harrowing account of being abandoned by her mother when she was a child, Johnson is not only able to contextualize her mother's behavior as a symptom of a sick society, but she bravely and lovingly assumes the responsibility of being her mother's sole caretaker. Yet Johnson consistently reminds us of the social and political responsibility that is denied to her mother. Although she picks up where society fails in caring for her mother, Johnson squarely lays blame "at the fault of society."

Vaquero and Salazar Vazquez bring forth both the domestic and global implications of the US immigration system's entanglement with racial capitalism. They show how this system accentuates the spread of COVID not only within US-based detention centers but transnationally through deportation.[14] Yet significantly, they do so while addressing the debilitating effects of carceral and punitive policies on immigrant families. Vaquero highlights that anti-immigration policies such as the public charge rule, which targets poorer immigrants who might depend on government assistant programs, did not begin with Trump but have much older roots in American policy. He also underscores the internalization of the false promise of the American dream, noting of his parents that, "Despite them having experienced blatant racism they continue to buy into this American dream that fails to take into account that we live under an umbrella of racial capitalism and white supremacy."[15] Vaquero situates racist immigration policies within the deeper foundation of racial capitalism—not only of the public charge rule or forced family separation, but more subtle forms of systemic racism that leaves his neighborhoods and communities affected by the pandemic in ways those with racialized immunoprivilege living in wealthier neighborhoods are not—to the deeper foundation of racial capitalism.

Salazar's powerful journal-entry format takes readers through a timeline that predates COVID. Beginning before the pandemic highlights how COVID does not create but rather exacerbates existing structural oppression. From his uncle's initial capture, there is already worry about the loss of his

financial contribution to sustaining the family. And then slowly, the intersections of ICE and the spread of COVID-19 are revealed. Poignantly, Salazar
Vazquez attributes his own COVID-19 infection to ICE and his uncle's deportation. From ICE agents not wearing masks, to overcrowding in detention
centers, to lack of resources for PPE for detainees, to transferring patients
between centers, and deporting infected people around the globe, Salazar
Vazquez illuminates through intimate details of his family's experience how
ICE perpetuated and exacerbated the pandemic.

Gutierrez provides an intersectional perspective on anti-Chinese hate and
structural racism experienced in New York's Chinatown. Due to the rise in
hate crimes toward people visibly racialized as East Asian, exacerbated by
former president Trump's anti-Chinese racist rhetoric, her piece speaks to an
increased public awareness and recognition of violence and racism toward
AAPI people. Gutierrez hints at the complexity involved in the racialization
of Asian-ness, being of mixed Dominican and Chinese descent herself. She
mentions on the one hand being alienated from her community by not being
accepted as Asian and presumed immune to anti-Asian hate. Yet she also
experienced anti-Asian racism from peers who assumed she was not Asian.
Her experience points to the contradiction of racialization as a process of
both interpellation and self-making.[16] On the one hand, a person's race is
determined by the state's interpellation of them, and the ways others thereby
treat them, and on the other, racialization is also a self-making process in
which racialized communities give meaning to their racial identity. However,
Guiterrez links interpersonal hate to the structural impacts of racism. She
notes that unemployment rose more among people of Asian descent than any
other racial group, that Asians are the most underrepresented racial group in
government leadership positions, and recounts the ways Chinatown and its
businesses were snubbed by NYC Mayor de Blasio, left without the support of
targeted government assistance to other racialized groups.[17]

Autoethnography as Witnessing

Writing about autoethnography, Stacy Holman Jones observes that "looking at the world from a specific, perspectival, and limited vantage point can
tell, teach and put people in motion."[18] She recounts an experience reading a
Carol Ronai essay in a graduate course. She explains how Ronai's language

and story "invited me into a lived felt experience. I could not stand outside of her words at safe remove. Ronai's story demanded that I respond and react."[19] Layla D. Brown-Vincent writes of her autoethnography, encountering, documenting, and analyzing the stories of Black Women and Afro-Venezuelan peoples as "an active attempt to make visible that which has been intentionally obscured by white supremacist patriarchal structures and institutions."[20] Yassir Morsi has written of his autoethnography as a "work of making visible my self-erasure" as a Muslim man and academic writing in the age of the Global War on Terror. "It cannot come through merely an analysis, it has to come from the lived experience."[21] In my teaching, I encourage students to embrace autoethnography, not only for the value their stories have for the world, but to instill in themselves the recognition of their own expertise, knowledge, and value of their own lived experience. I seek to use anti-racist, feminist pedagogy to counteract structural racism in our educational system that too often teaches our students to disregard that which they already know—to disregard their inherent knowledge and possibilities for collective power.

In my teaching, research, and personal experiences, I am particularly attuned to the racialized subjugation of Muslims under white supremacy. In my final year of graduate school, I taught the same course, titled Racializing Muslims, at both The New School (TNS), where I was completing my doctoral studies, and as an adjunct at Brooklyn College. The intersectional inequality between the two student populations and the discrepancy between positionality and knowledge, was brought into stark relief. At TNS there were no Muslim students in the class, whereas at Brooklyn College all save one student was Muslim. At Brooklyn most of my students had a number of external obligations that infringed upon their time outside of class, such as full-time jobs and family responsibilities. Some explained that they often didn't have time to complete assignments unless it was something they could do while at work. TNS students rarely had outside jobs and many lived in the campus dorms. Yet despite relative structural disadvantages, my students at Brooklyn had an experiential knowledge of the racialization of Muslims that impacted the class both in terms of the knowledge they brought into the classroom space and in terms of my own objectives as a teacher. My Brooklyn students didn't need to be educated that the category of Muslim is a racialized category—they lived that reality. What I saw as my pedagogical task was to provide a language for them to describe, analyze, and understand that which they already knew. During his presentation, one student at BC shared a clip from an *Ironman* movie in which the protagonist uses a special device in his suit to separate the terrorist Muslims from the "good" Muslims being held hostage, instantaneously killing the former while saving the latter. The clip brilliantly exemplified Mahmood Mamdani's argument in "Good Muslim, Bad Muslim"[22] about a racialized war on terror that creates a binary in which Muslims must prove themselves worthy before being considered human. In another example, toward the end of the semester a group of young women in the Brooklyn class shared with me their frustrations with a meeting with the then newly appointed president of the college in a "listening session" as part of the administration's "We Stand Against Hate" Campaign. The young women complained that when they recounted instances of assault—multiple women had reported their hijabs being pulled off while on campus—the administration proposed no resolutions and made no calls for systemic change. The women told me that they felt "used" as if part of a promotional stunt, without their experiences being taken seriously. This disconnect between normalized structural oppression, experienced and understood by marginalized people, and a liberal, performative, so-called "anti-racism" that upholds the status quo of existing structural conditions, catalyzed activist organizers at Brooklyn College during the pandemic.

As the pandemic, BLM uprising, and student autoethnographies in this collection inspired demands for revolutionary change, at Brooklyn College I was among a group of students, staff, and faculty who also rose to challenge the entrenched racial hierarchies that are reproduced on our campus. Amid the uprising in May 2020 members of the Black Faculty and Staff Group drafted a statement calling out the particularity of anti-blackness and how it manifested at Brooklyn College.[23] The letter asked us all to imagine what a Black-life-affirming campus would look like. Calling out the administration's empty stand against "hate," the letter and all those who endorsed it recognized that while racism in the form of individualized and personalized hate was *also* a problem on campus, it paled in comparison to accepted and unacknowledged forms of institutionalized racism. The letter addressed years of purposeful inaction[24] on the part of administration to support Black students, address the dwindling number of already minimal Black faculty, and the overrepresentation of Black employees in subordinate and precarious staff positions—all at a campus with over 20% Black students[25] that is situated at the intersections of a predominantly Black Caribbean neighborhood. The activist student group the Puerto Rican Alliance also addressed a letter to the college president, highlighting years of structural racism in the forms of underfunding Black, Indigenous, and Latinx programs, departments, and students. Following a dismissive response from the president, in conjunction with union organizing against ongoing austerity measures putting precarious lives at further risk, a coalition of students, staff, and faculty formed the Anti-Racist Coalition (ARC) at Brooklyn College.[26]

ARC promoted a materialist and structural analysis of racism. Our first event was a student-led Town Hall highlighting the lived experience of structural racism on campus. The students, staff, and faculty who made up ARC foregrounded that we already knew how to confront inequality on our campus. We didn't need to go outside to solve the issues of structural racism on our campus. We simply needed a governing body that would listen—would take seriously the knowledge carried by our students, staff, and faculty as we confront structural racism every day on our own campus. With testimonials from a queer Black student recounting their difficulties obtaining transfer credits, causing them to have to prolong their studies despite financial hardship; a working mother who phoned in from the bus on her way to work; a Muslim student detailing the continued effects of police surveillance; and others, students articulated their experiences in terms of structural conditions. They recognized that not all students were given the same opportunities and that those inequalities were structurally racist. Connecting white supremacy to racial capitalism, and making the link between austerity and structural racism, ARC was a product of the 2020 uprising. We built upon the analysis of structural racism provided by BLM—one that serves as a model for non-Black marginalized groups. Instead of pitting differently racialized communities against each other, an analysis of intersecting logics of white supremacy[27] allows for the recognition of intersectional exploitation. Recognizing the only liberation is collective liberation, Tobago-born Canadian poet and essayist M. NourbeSe Philip stated early on in the pandemic: "Were we truly 'in this together,' we would not be in 'this' together."[28]

One of the most powerful outcomes of the 2020 uprising was the mainstreaming of calls for transformational, structural change. When longtime prison abolitionist organizer Mariame Kaba was published in the *New York Times*, abolition entered mainstream discourse, and several cities across the country passed reforms to defund the police and redistribute resources to life-affirming public institutions.[29] At the time of writing this, three years in, the pandemic is not over. Mask-mandates have been lifted yet the virus has not been eliminated. Potential remains for new variants to emerge and the effects and repercussions of long COVID are yet to be known.[30]

The student autoethnographies in this collection incite us to confront society as structured according to the logic of white supremacy under racial capitalism. These moments and stories force us to see how the organization of our world sacrifices the majority to further the profits of an increasingly small elite capitalist class. I often remind my students to remember that white supremacy is not the shark, it is the water.[31] Instead of accepting white supremacy's ubiquity as impenetrable, its ubiquity means that we have opportunity to dismantle it in nearly every facet of our lives. Fortified with stories portraying the lived experience of state-organized abandonment under racial capitalism, may we collectively refuse the white supremacist status quo that has dominated the planet for over five hundred years. May we enact a new world that centers, uplifts, and affirms Billie-Rae Johnson's mother, Anthony Salazar Vazquez's uncle, Raúl Vaquero's parents, Kayla Gutierrez's grandmother, and all the other voices and lives that "normality" has attempted to render invisible.

PART III

Crises of Health and Housing

CHAPTER 11

America's Health Care System Needs 911

Anthony Almojera

"Conditions 4-0 for the assignment. Conditions 4-0, take it over to Sixty-Eighth Street and Fourth Avenue for the unconscious. Twenty-seven-year-old found unresponsive by mother. No other details," the dispatch radio cackles. "Conditions 40" is my call sign. It means I work in the 40th Emergency Medical Services (EMS) battalion, which covers much of what was called South Brooklyn in the old days, including the neighborhoods of Sunset Park, Bay Ridge, and Dyker Heights. I pick up the mic and say with a degree of wariness, "Conditions 4-0, show me en route." The pandemic has taken its toll on us medics, and we were all suffering with a degree of PTSD. I put my command vehicle in drive and turned on the lights and sirens.

I arrive on scene and the ambulance with the medics pulls up right in front of me. I nod and start to get my equipment, as they get theirs. I put my N-95 mask on and grab extra gloves. It's a five-story walkup and of course the patient is on the fifth floor. The sickest people are always on the top floors of the old tenements; it's economics, but more on that later. We get up the stairs with all our equipment and the mother is yelling for us to hurry. We can hear by her voice it's serious—there's nothing like the scream of a parent when their kid is genuinely sick. That sound gets in your bones as a medic and never gets out. We walk in and there's a kid or what looks like a kid on the floor, not breathing and no pulse. I kneel and he is extremely cold and stiff; he has dependent lividity, which is when the blood pools at the lowest point in the body. It also means there is nothing we can do for him. Here is the part that is getting tougher for me as the years march on: I have to tell the mom he's dead and we can't help him. If this were a ninety-year-old man dying of old age or a person in a freak accident, it would be easier. We can rationalize those, but it is hard to wrap your head around the death of a twenty-seven-year-old. After I ask the mom for some more information about what was going on with him, it gets worse. His mother states he is a type 1 diabetic and lost his health insurance this year due to the pandemic. He was working, but didn't have a job that provided health insurance or paid him enough to buy his insulin outright. He died from rationing his insulin, which is deadly for a diabetic.

During the pandemic there were many patients who suffered or died in similar circumstances. They were what a soldier would call collateral damage. The Centers for Disease Control reports that in 2020, 31.6 million Americans were uninsured. Of that number, 27.5 million were between the ages of twenty-one and sixty-five.[1] Obamacare did not go far enough in guaranteeing health care coverage for all. It merely set up exchanges for insurance companies to make greater profits and offer health plans that did not cover or cover enough for people who needed medical insurance. These numbers do not account for undocumented immigrant populations, which studies have shown tend to live in metropolitan areas. Combine these numbers with those large cities where adequate housing is scarce and expensive, leading to multiple generations living in one household, and you have the perfect setup for a pandemic to wreak havoc. While over eighty thousand people have died from COVID in New York City since the outset of the pandemic, the collateral deaths—deaths from lack of health care—take the number far higher.[2] The fact that in the world's richest country scenes like the young man dying of diabetes take place daily, and have been exacerbated by the COVID-19 pandemic, is a stain on our American souls.

My name is Anthony Almojera. I am forty-six years old and was born and raised in Brooklyn, New York. I am a paramedic lieutenant for the Fire Department of New York (FDNY) Emergency Medical Service (EMS) command, and I received my undergraduate degree from Brooklyn College in 2021. I have been working the streets of New York City for twenty years. I started my career doing medical transport, not necessarily answering 911 calls, but helping sick people get to their appointments and home from their surgeries. It was that year and a half prior to being hired by the FDNY when I started to hear the horror stories of what our medical system does to the average person. When I say average, I am talking about middle to lower class economically, regular working folks who had the misfortune to get sick in a country that practices medical capitalism. They would tell me stories of having to declare bankruptcy to pay for nursing homes or take out second mortgages to pay back medical debt. We would see this amplified during the pandemic: millions of people lost their jobs with no social safety net to help keep them afloat; businesses shut down, and people could not make mortgage and rent payments; people lost the ability to pay for health insurance or drugs they need to stay alive.

This was not the first time I had experienced these health inequities. In 2003, my father went into liver failure. He had developed hepatitis C, a death sentence at the time unless a new liver was available. He was a longshoreman and had a good job with what I thought were good benefits. Growing up, I was able to see doctors and we never lacked for routine medical care. Therefore, I was shocked to find out that a liver transplant was estimated to cost close to $1 million when you consider surgery, medications, and rehab. I was new to the medical field, and this was an eye-opening experience. His medical insurance would only cover up to $300,000. My father was told if he had Medicaid, it would almost cover it all, but because of his salary and owning a home, he was ineligible. They told him he would have to quit his job, declare bankruptcy, and maybe then he would qualify for Medicaid. I was with him when he received this news. His face is imprinted in my memory like a frozen screen saver, a complete look of anger and dejection. It would be a face I would see time and again working as a paramedic.

In 2004, after I had worked medical transport for a couple of years, the FDNY finally called. I was ready to take the next step and respond to 911 emergencies. I was assigned to Harlem right out of the academy, and I loved it! It was busy, my coworkers were great, and the neighborhood, filled with so much history, was fascinating. This wasn't the currently gentrifying Harlem; it was still reeling from years of a drug epidemic. I was responding to some of the craziest calls of my life, but there was a common thread with my old job back in transport: so many people without medical insurance or the basics to support a healthy life. I would respond to calls where people would wait until the last minute with their heart or asthma attacks. When you have sizable parts of the population with little to no actual access to primary medical care, people with limited means will be forced to prioritize what they need to survive. The nagging high blood pressure will go by the wayside to put food on the table for the kids. The medical conditions neglected over the years would act like dry kindling in a drought when a pandemic comes along, the virus taking advantage of a body that has been neglected by a system designed to monetize sickness instead of wellness. Rather than providing stabilizing care, we were asked to become primary care providers and reverse end-of-life diseases.

In my FDNY career I worked all over New York City, including Harlem, the South Bronx, East Flatbush, Midtown Manhattan, and Sunset Park. I have walked into mansions and have responded to homeless shelters, but the overwhelming majority of people who call 911 are people without primary access to medical care. They use the emergency rooms as their primary care physicians. This is equivalent to using duct tape for everything broken. The medical systems I was operating in, including EMS, were set up to maximize profit over patients. America's medical system is a house of cards that was just waiting for a stiff wind to blow it over.

The emergency medical services are reflections of the sick society we respond to. Years of mismanagement and underfunding have left us with a permanently revolving door. Seventy-five percent of FDNY EMS have five years or less experience; when I was hired, it was seventeen years' experience. EMS is currently 58% minority and 38% women. We are the most diverse 911 workforce. On average firefighters and cops make approximately $35,000 dollars more than paramedics. This is in spite of us responding to 1.9 million calls, as opposed to approximately 54,000 fire runs. There are only about four thousand EMS members, while there are around eleven thousand firefighters and over thirty thousand police officers. The disparity in personnel and money has led to the erosion of morale and overall workforce. Back in 2008 a federal judge found the FDNY in violation of racial hiring practices and forced the department to make it easier for minorities and women to become firefighters. This lawsuit by the FDNYs Vulcan society did nothing, however, to address EMS and our long-standing issues. It actually made them worse, as the FDNY looked to its EMS workforce to fill its ranks with the people to address this mandate. EMS regularly loses twelve hundred people on average to firefighting classes through an intra-department exam geared to give EMS people first crack at being hired. This further weakens our ranks and accelerates the brain drain of experienced medics.

The less than robust benefits make working for EMS a challenge. We have EMTs who collect public assistance and a majority are forced to work two and three jobs. We also only get twelve sick days a year. Compare that to firefighters, sanitation workers, and police officers who all get unlimited sick leave. The people who take care of sick people only get twelve days a year.

Once we burn through those days, we can fall off payroll, and when that happens, we lose our medical insurance. The fund-raising site GoFundMe has become a default medical insurance for EMS members; often we must chip in to make sure medics can remain financially solvent when they are sick long term. When you're charged with saving lives for a living, that should be the only job you need to do to be able to live comfortably.

For years EMS has floated along like this—a patchwork of different entities trying to put together a 911 response system. There have been numerous times where I thought we would break. The big blizzards, power outages, and various other natural and manmade events bent us but surprisingly we did not crack. It's a real testament to the men and women who work this job that we were able to weather those events with relatively few negative outcomes.

My personal life started to reflect the job I was working. My dad did eventually get a new liver, which bought him another ten years, but he passed in 2012. My mother followed in 2013. She wound up in a nursing home which bled her dry financially. I was in my own financial rut. Having taken out student loans along with the debt incurred taking care of sick parents and funeral expenses, I had to drop out of college. I made numerous attempts to finish college, a journey I started back in 2000, but kept having to withdraw. My personal relationships suffered. There was no time, as I was becoming more enmeshed with EMS, running for union delegate positions, and having to work three jobs and overtime to be able to make ends meet. In 2017 I decided to recommit and try and get my degree. I had already invested so much time and money. I went part-time to complete my studies and I eventually did get on a roll in school and was scheduled to graduate in the fall of 2020. Then the pandemic hit. I was not able to attend classes when the outbreak first happened. Work was too busy, and school had shut down. When school started to offer the classes online in the fall of 2020, I was able to attend. It was a reprieve for me. In the winter of 2020 I was home recovering from surgery for a work-related injury, and I found a sense of community in my classes. School gave me something to look forward to and helped abate the loneliness of being isolated through the multiple waves of COVID. I eventually graduated from Brooklyn College with my degree in Political Science in the spring of 2021.

The house of cards that America's health care system and its emergency medical services are built on would eventually get tested like never before. Around October 2019 a new virus was reported by the Centers for Disease Control. It was called SAR-CoV-1, later to be known as COVID-19.

My station is located in Brooklyn's Chinatown. In its confines lives the borough's largest concentration of Chinese immigrants. When the virus first appeared, we started to alert members at roll call about it. We gave a brief synopsis of the virus and reminded the members that there are direct flights from the affected regions to New York City. We have been through epidemics before. We had SARS and even a couple of Ebola patients, and I thought that this would mirror those outbreaks. The protocols in place basically treated a patient as you would in a hazardous materials incident. We would suit up in thick Tyvek suits, multiple gloves, and an escape mask, which looks like a gas mask and operates similarly. When we had the Ebola patient, the call got two ambulances and a fire engine to treat the patient and decontaminate the ambulance and crews. The FDNY essentially stated that with COVID-19 we would follow the same protocols. We thought early on that this would be okay. However, when we saw the speed at which it spread through Italy and the number of patients they were reporting, we realized there would be serious issues with trying to treat everyone like our Ebola patient. In late January 2020, I testified in front of the New York City Council about this. I stated that EMS needs to be fully funded and staffed to handle anything that may come along and tax the 911 medical system. The FDNY representatives on scene, which included the Chief of EMS Lillian Bonsignore, testified that EMS was fine in its current state and ready for anything. Those words would soon come back to haunt them.

On March 20, 2020, the EMS equivalent of the Hiroshima bomb dropped. A few days prior to that we started to get COVID calls coming into the 911 system and the call volume started to rise. During normal operations there are approximately 3500–4,000 EMS calls daily in New York City. The mayor in the weeks prior to March 20 went on television to tell everyone to continue to go to restaurants and theatres. We in EMS thought this was terrible advice and started to ring the alarm on the station level. The FDNY brass, though, was remarkably silent; no real plans other than treat and make notifications. On March 20, the call volume spiked to over 5,000 calls, on March 24 to 6,406, on March 25 to 6,550, and on March 26 to 7,111. Just to give you some context, on 9/11 we had about 6,500 calls come into EMS but there weren't 6,500 patients; many of those calls were people calling multiple times to try to find family and friends. As one doctor in Bellevue stated, "We were open, but nobody showed up." This was the complete opposite: over 7,000 calls to EMS and they were all patients. This went on for over two months.

As the city exploded with COVID cases, EMS started to fracture. We started to get sick. At one point over one-quarter of our workforce was out sick with COVID. Many members were hospitalized and sent to already over-crowded ICUs. The ancillary effect of all of this was there were 911 calls not being answered. We simply did not have the personnel for it. Then some of us started to die from COVID. At the time of this writing, ten members have passed away and numerous others have not been able to come back to work. The hospitals had lines around the corner. They started to run out of ventila-tors and staff. The proverbial house of cards that we call America's health care system started to collapse.

According to a CNBC personal finance report dated August 12, 2020, up to 12 million people lost their employer-based health insurance during the initial wave of the pandemic.[3] As employers closed or furloughed work-ers, people who were living on the financial margins were not able to afford medical insurance like COBRA and others offered on the exchanges. The government had not provided any type of financial relief; nor did it man-date insurance companies to continue with their coverage for an extended period after job loss. As an example, if an EMS FDNY employee falls off payroll due to running out of sick time, their medical insurance is canceled within twenty-four hours of that date. As the pandemic wore on, we started to go to calls where people had delayed calling 911 or getting to their per-sonal doctors. According to a study by the Reason Foundation, by September of 2020 there were more than 20,000 deaths above the normal seasonal rate outside of reported COVID deaths.[4] The study attributed the excess deaths to poverty, lost jobs, and lack of access to health care and medical insurance. This study states that the numbers of collateral deaths over the coming years will continue to rise through subsequent waves of COVID variants and the gaps in preventative care and monitoring will have a lasting impact on health. I went on numerous calls with people who delayed getting treated because they lost their jobs. They lost their health insurance in the middle of a global pandemic! I responded to a person having chest pain for four days. He stated he lost his health insurance and was hoping the pain would resolve on its own. When the medics checked him out, he was having a major heart attack. By the time they got to the hospital, they were doing CPR. Another call was a fifty-eight-year-old woman who lost her job in a Manhattan office build-ing doing maintenance work. She had been receiving therapy for a stroke she suffered a few years back. When she lost her job, she lost the medical insurance that was paying for the therapy along with it. I remember her saying the out-of-pocket expense would be $400 a session. Her conditions had deteriorated, and she hadn't taken the necessary blood pressure medications for the same reasons. We took her blood pressure, and it was 200/110. She stated she did not know what else to do and tried to wait for the pandemic to subside, but the headaches were getting worse. She was isolating for fear of contracting COVID, but now we had to take her to a hospital that was overrun with COVID patients. The pandemic destroyed the thin threads that so many people were holding onto trying to make it through life—many of them poor and disenfranchised people to begin with. The man with chest pains did not make it. It seems my medical career has gone full circle.

For twenty years I have been responding to 911 calls in New York City. These experiences have allowed me to be more empathetic and sympathetic to the patients I treat. But we are up against a system of greed and apathy—one where human beings are discarded in the name of corporate profits. The very fact that more than twelve million people lost their health insurance during a pandemic that has killed over a million Americans and there have been no fundamental changes is a tragedy in of itself.

We in EMS were used as sacrificial pawns, expendable to the city. We will carry the burden of what we have seen for the rest of our lives. Not all of us are able to do so; since the beginning of the pandemic, there have been eight suicides in the FDNY EMS command. The inequalities were laid bare. We live in and take care of this city. For us, there was no hiding from COVID-19. We did not have the luxury of clapping at hospitals like the firefighters did to show support for medical staff; the sound of banging pots and pans were drowned out by our sirens. I remember reading during this time that the housing market was on fire. People with financial means were in the market to acquire second and third homes in far-flung places to escape the pandemic and live in comfortable isolation. EMS workers can barely afford the places they live in now. We were mirroring the patients we were taking care of, the ones left behind. The rich went to the Hamptons, the poor and uninsured were sent to their graves.

CHAPTER 12

What It Means to Be an Anxious Pakistani During a Global Pandemic

Areeba Zanub

i remember the sky being so blue and the sun being so bright

12,
i awaken in recovery position, a bright light emerges from darkness.
my science teacher hovers over me: *you fainted, it's going to be okay.*
this   can't   be   happening   right   now   i hyperventilate
at the hospital, a doctor makes me follow a light: *you had an anxiety
    attack.*
my parents, impatient: *the ambulance. the emergency room. this is
    going to cost us.*

15,
i awaken, stunned by bright classroom lights. my head throbs.
my math teacher kneels beside me: *we heard a loud bang, and here
    you are on the floor! we called the nurse.*
this can't be happening   not right now
i help myself up, i hear a laugh, i hyperventilate
and.it.happens.all.over.again.
the nurse walks in, guiding a wheelchair: *do you want me to call your
    parents?*
my lips part: *no, i just need a few minutes to calm down.*
i skip class the next day.

a week later,
my doctor refers me to a cardiologist; i mentioned that my heart was
      racing.
at the appointment, a medical intern speaks first: *do you ever feel
      lonely? or nervous?*
i don't know how to reply, no one has ever asked me this
      before.
i think of the hospital bills: *no, and no.*
the final verdict from dr. cardiologist: *nothing is wrong with your
      heart. things like this*
*happen—maybe it was because the scarf on your head made you feel
      hot and you fainted from*
a hot flash? still, nothing is wrong with your heart.
in the car, my mom: *they don't know anything about us, we shouldn't
      have gone.*

16,
inside the mosque, i pray. i shake as i rise from total submission,
and then as i contemplate my existence,
i collapse
and everything suddenly becomes dark all at once.
a brown woman in black chador, picks me up: *where is your mom?*
i say: *i don't know, i think just had an anxiety attack.*
she: *anxiety? at this age? over what? oh no, darling, you are too young
      to be having anxiety.*

18,
on campus, in an elevator, alone.
i'm beginning to believe that
i.am.being.closed.in
i imagine the elevator falling. no one can hear my screams.
i   can't   breathe.   please.
it opens, *thank God.*
i run to the first floor   onto the field   towards the campus bench
      but the darkness follows
and then i awaken again.
and the sun's rays hit my eyes.

a week later,
at the community doctor's office.
i admire the Pakistani flag above the height chart. i feel safe.
my mom leaves the room so i can speak to *dr. community* alone.
i say: *i am struggling. i often convince myself that i am dying, i know i
    am not but once the thought emerges, it really feels like it.*
dr. community laughs: *get out of your head, it'll be over by your twen-
    ties. by the way, you are missing a few vaccines.*

*   *   *

I looked out of our apartment window and watched a woman wearing a surgical mask rush down the street. I had just finished my morning prayers when my mom came beside me, holding prayer beads, anxiously awaiting my dad's return home from work. We could hear sirens from afar as the sun began to rise and when the doorbell rang, she practically jumped. Before my dad could even step inside, my mom sprayed various antiseptics down to his shoes while he updated her about the new cases.

A couple of weeks had passed since the lockdown began. COVID-19 was plastered on every news outlet while surgical masks littered the streets. Grocery store shelves stood emptied out. It was eerily apocalyptic, yet it had already been dubbed the "new normal."

I was diagnosed with agoraphobia and generalized anxiety disorder a few months before. I would wish—*beg*—for days when I could just hide away from the world and not have to fight to live anymore.

Now, the same isolation that I prayed for suffocated me.

I felt like I was drowning in the walls of my own room. The lack of connection resulted in days that blended and blurred. The death tolls, the sirens, the uncertainty—the days darkened before they even began as the media only showed the pandemic worsening.

The day our landlord died from COVID was extremely difficult. He was close to our family and not long after he passed, his father decided to sell the building. We were financially drowning and struggling to find a new apartment due to the housing shortage. My dad couldn't risk working due to his severe asthma and my mom was strict on staying home. Our family's financial situation had been bad before, but the pandemic was a new playing field. It seemed there was no room for consolation.

My lowest moment during the height of the pandemic was a desperation for communication—to speak, interact, even *touch*. I secretly clung to the free therapy offered at CUNY, but with no in-person services available, my anxiety became restless. I was lost and without support.

As a Pakistani-American, I had always been met with indifference by members of my own community regarding my mental health—psychological and emotional invalidation, backhanded advice, subtle disregard, or simple ignorance. Outward displays of mental disorders were simply unacceptable.

I became desperate to unfold my community's struggle with mental health stigma. It was during the pandemic that I realized that a first step to confronting my own mental health issues meant understanding that it had a larger context in the history of the people around me—the Pakistani community.

My community had always been where I first searched for comfort and validation: I saw mosques filled with hugs and kisses, gatherings filled with the benevolence of strangers who despite not knowing each other, knew each other. Community was more than an assembly of people—it was a lived experience, an unbroken chain of Desi culture, music, love, language, and art. We were a family, bound by the same national roots and all congregated in a foreign land, trying to make a home. We understood each other's struggles and we shared similar stories of Pakistan and immigrating to New York.

My people are strong—they have endured the pain and suffering of partition, immigration, economic struggle, and loss, and came out of it alive. Still, I felt there was something missing in our conversations about resilience: the proper awareness, acknowledgment, or even the simple recognition of mental health—I'm speaking about the unspoken.

I'm speaking about the countless number of Pakistani children whose mental health has gone unnoticed or who have been neglected, who've been left undiagnosed and then untreated.

I'm speaking about the countless number of Pakistani women who were abused for years under their own roof, the same ones who were neglected and shamed, who were told to stay quiet because *what will people say*?

I'm speaking about the countless number of Pakistani fathers, homesick and lonely in their empty American apartments, counting the days until their wife and children are granted visas, the same ones who were told that tears on a man are a sign of weakness.

I'm speaking about the older generation, the ones who fled during the 1947 British India Partition, the ones who witnessed massacres, rape, and famine, the ones who didn't process trauma in their lifetimes amid all the fight for their land and freedom, the ones who were forced to live with it and then struggled to explain their sorrow to their children.

I'm speaking about this because it is bigger than my own mental health being disregarded. This experience of generational trauma and mental health stigma extends across and even beyond Pakistani communities.

When examining COVID-19 through a framework of BIPOC and immigrant mental health, it becomes clear that the heightened rates of mortality, the uncertainty, the political powerlessness, the economic collapse, and the struggle to effectively cope with these issues are impacting us more deeply. The fears and threats posed by COVID-19 intersect with the history our community carries. As a consequence, we are dealing with both present and generational trauma.

The conversation about death is not new for us, but the acceptance of and need for allowing grief is. The conversation about mental health is new, but the denial isn't.

In fact, the denial is deeply rooted in culture. That was the disconnect that led me back to where I started—Pakistan, when the opportunity to visit after ten years arose later in 2021.

Seeing the vast green fields and old salt ranges posed against the withered faces of elders, carrying all that history, all that trauma, moved me. We've been here a long time.

Borders ruled our land and the violence that came with the Partition no doubt set a stage for a history of PTSD, depression, and grief.

I sought out my elders who were alive before 1947, before the Islamic Republic of Pakistan existed. They spoke about Pakistan being forged in a fight for self-determination. Individual thought, freedom, opinions, and emotion were often sacrificed for the sake of political and civil development. We neglected our own trauma and as time passed, it became one of our biggest barriers—to speak about our mental health without stigmatizing it.

The elders I spoke with acknowledged that the trauma of the war is to blame for the loneliness and restlessness experienced by today's youth which undid the common practice of gathering in one place and expressing their feelings of joy and sorrow together.

Yet, I quickly discovered that seeking mental health treatment in Pakistan is subject to scrutiny and stigma. Avoiding emotions and swallowing the pain became a survival technique for our ancestors, whose history is marked by economic and social resettlement, bloody warfare, and destruction. More-over, the pressure and culturally normative expectations of socioeconomic prosperity for immigrants upon their arrival in the United States hindered subsequent generations from addressing their pain.

In a culture oriented toward survival and determination, discussing mental health issues is perceived as a sign of weakness and runs contrary to an expected display of strength. This perception is so prevalent that it is often not recognized as a problem.

Stigma discredits lived experience through silence, thus complicating it as the stigmatized individual begins to avoid confronting their own pain. Consequently, this stigma prolongs the duration of mental health disorders by preventing individuals from seeking treatment or acknowledging the significance of their mental health. As a result, trauma is continuously passed down, reproducing the same disparities as the elder generation, feeding into the cycle of silence and repression.

Although generational trauma in the Pakistani community is unique to the nation's history, it also reflects a broader pattern. Generational trauma finds itself buried in BIPOC and immigrant communities all across the United States. The pandemic only furthered our already-present emotional and mental health challenges while simultaneously calling attention to the structurally racist histories of wellness systems, which are driven by conscious and unconscious racial biases, lack of inclusivity, and unaffordability.[1]

Due to socioeconomic factors such as immigration, limited access to health care, unemployment, discrimination, and generational trauma, BIPOC communities persistently encounter obstacles related to mental health. These preexisting circumstances were only made worse by COVID-19's socioeconomic impact[2] as BIPOC and immigrants faced a devastating increase in mortality and unemployment rates during the pandemic.[3] Therefore, we became more susceptible to the physiological, social, political, and economic repercussions of that followed. Our communities suffered a higher prevalence of psychopathology rates as a result.[4] For this reason, we cannot have a singular approach to mental health care as different cultural groups have specific needs and experiences that reflect their unique histories. In order to address these differences, it's essential to be more inclusive, culturally sensitive, and trauma informed.

A lot of time has passed since lockdown and turning back to the present, I am hopeful. I've felt the presence of collectivism—the same presence that our ancestors felt throughout their period of survival. As everyone experienced loss during the pandemic, grief and anxiety have become acceptable topics of discourse. This threat to humanity's well-being highlighted the significance of mental health—a long-ignored concern that is now even more critical to acknowledge, especially in light of all of the mourning associated with the pandemic.

A sign of promise for mental health care is the growing use of technology and video-chatting services like Zoom and Google Meets to establish safe spaces for therapy and support groups. Additionally, young people are taking control of their own mental health treatment by using online forums to express their concerns and sympathize with one another. Individuals have taken the effort to form inclusive networks for those who are experiencing mental health difficulties like frontline workers and marginalized communities. Even CUNY Mental Health Services made remarkable progress by developing online tools like Kognito, 10 Minute Mind, and partnering with Crisis Text Line to assist students in need of mental health support, guide them to appropriate services, and aid them in managing stressful situations off campus. Personally, I found Togetherall an excellent tool for receiving anonymous support and alleviating my own emotions of loneliness without having to worry about shame or affordability.

On the other side of the world in Pakistan, action is being taken by coalitions like Taskeen[5] and the British Asian Trust,[6] who are striving to change the mental health landscape by increasing consciousness, destigmatizing mental disorders, and advocating for readily available mental health care. A hopeful transformation is being pushed across the country whose resources for mental health are insufficient. These two partners, as well as many others, are motivated to improve systems and, in particular, change attitudes. A clear shift in the public perception can be seen in the exchange and embrace of memories of the 1947 British India Partition.[7] Oral histories being uncovered show how urgent the need for constructive dialogue and depiction of South Asia's past and collective awareness is in order to break the cycle of silence.

These coalitions especially stepped up during COVID-19 by offering mental health care to frontline workers and others in Pakistan who were directly impacted by the pandemic. These groups encouraged community-based mental health services in primary health care settings and schools, expanded education, and advocated for structural and legislative changes.

In light of the tremendous suffering and anxiety caused by the pandemic, the opportunity it has given us for understanding and solidarity among people is great.

This is a starting place—to recognize the discrepancies and particular issues we encounter as marginalized people by sharing our experiences.

In this same regard, we must press for more community resources, therapeutic facilities, and systems of care that are affordable, diverse, take into account local contexts like family, socioeconomic issues, and immigration. These would allow us to collectively share our experiences without stigma and shame, and strengthen our social connectedness in a time of fear, loneliness, and struggle. Although intentionally inclusive therapeutic spaces exist, which are culturally responsive and acknowledge privilege and Eurocentric biases that may arise in the treatment of BIPOC patients,[8] the majority of therapeutic spaces lack this cultural attunement. The standard for mental health care should prioritize affordability and cultural inclusivity instead of uniformity. It is only then that we can move away from stigma and combat the worldviews that developed from our unprocessed generational trauma—the silencing, the lack of trust, the repression of pain, the need to be continuously strong, and the invalidation of anything less than strong.

Presently, I am writing from Islamabad, the capital of Pakistan. My life is split in two: I am here, yet my family and friends are in New York City. Still, despite being in an entirely different environment, nothing seems unfamiliar. Fatima Asghar puts it better, "My country is made in my people's image." The essence of Pakistan is made by my people's collective efforts—our history, our rich culture, our fight for freedom.

I could write about the lush green landscapes I've seen, the forts I've climbed, the clear waters I've drunk from, the exhilarating stories I've heard, but I want to tell you about the most beautiful thing I've seen since visiting: a funeral.

I was sitting on a divan at our ancestral home, reading, when I heard the news of my mother's aunt's passing. She was an elderly woman who faced a lot of hardship through her life, living through the Partition and economic struggle, yet her charisma pierced through everyone who got to know her.

At the funeral, memories of the past were traded like sweets and a powerful sense of collective resilience shifted amid the pandemic's darkness. I had never seen anything like the process of community mourning I saw during this time. Strength was found in remembrance, and communicating those joyous memories was what kept these families moving forward.

In the depths of what seemed like a dark time, the brightness was the realization that no amount of tragedy could sever the strong bonds we had forged and rooted in years of collective struggle, but only bring us closer.

I can only anticipate how much more we'll bloom.

CHAPTER 13

Livin' in the Projects: COVID-19 and Community Resilience

Dominick Braswell

May 15, 2020

It is a little over two months into the COVID-19 pandemic and my community has been completely disrupted. As I walk through the Albany Housing Projects, which I call home, it is an eerily silent and desolate scene. What would ordinarily be a Friday buzzing with life and activity is the opposite. The playground outside of the children's daycare center, which would typically be occupied by screaming and laughing toddlers, is devoid of their presence. Our community center would normally be filled with elderly residents taking computer classes and kids working on homework after school, but now it sits vacant, lights off, and doors locked. The benches in the outdoor common area, usually filled with neighbors playing music and gossiping, are empty. Ms. Angela and our building watch team are absent from the table in the lobby where they normally play cards and keep an eye on incoming and outgoing traffic. The pandemic has suspended life as usual in my neighborhood.

Due to the health risk, we could no longer gather to perform many of the ritualistic community bonding practices we had grown accustomed to at Albany Houses. COVID had shifted life for many of us here at the housing complex. For the first two years of the pandemic, unless you were going out for groceries or you were an essential worker, most people stayed sheltered in their apartments. According to a New York City Housing Authority (NYCHA) demographic sheet, 40.8% of the city's public housing units are headed by residents aged sixty-two or older.[1] That same study also found that the annual income of the average public housing family was $24,503.[2] Thirty-four percent of Albany Houses' 2,700 residents live on a fixed income.[3] Because the elderly are particularly vulnerable to contracting the virus, and because preexisting health conditions such as asthma are common among low-income communities of color, most of us who live in Albany Houses, and public housing more generally, are at a heightened risk of deadly contraction of the virus.[4] This fact made my neighbors and me even more anxious and fearful. Yet we were used to living under, and having to adjust to, difficult conditions. As tenants of an old and dilapidated public housing complex, we have persistently dealt with rodent and roach infestations, old leaky pipes, mold, and heatless winters due to a boiler that often breaks. These issues are the result of decades of neglect by state and federal officials. We have routinely had to organize to pressure NYCHA to deal with building maintenance and other concerns when they were slow or unwilling. The same has unfortunately been true for us during the pandemic—and despite the risks, the very community that came together in times of leisure has also come together to aid each other in the time of COVID-19.

I chose to open this narrative with a description of how COVID-19 impacted my housing complex as a community because in the last fifty-plus years of popular discourse surrounding public housing in America, the word *community* has often been omitted in illustrations of life in the projects. What we have received instead from popular news media are horrific and disastrous depictions of public housing developments that are more like violent battlefronts than actual communities. Chicago's the *Daily Northwestern* published an article in 2000 titled "Chicago Public Housing: The Worst Place in the Country," which opens by telling readers that if you live in the projects "you're twice as likely to be shot" than in other working-class neighborhoods.[5] Researcher Lynn Olson is quoted in the piece describing life within public housing as "equivalent to growing up in a war zone."[6] In 2019, the *Brooklyn Eagle* published an article titled "At NYCHA's Most Dangerous Development, Tenants Wonder: Is the City Doing Enough?" about tenants at NYCHA's Bushwick Houses not feeling safe due to a double homicide that took place there a year before.[7] Speaking about how unsafe she felt after the murders, a resident named Dominique is quoted saying, "I want to get the fuck out of here."[8] In 2019 the *New York Post* published an article, "NYCHA Crime Surges as Harlem's Wagner Houses Become Gang Battleground," about a 15% increase in crime at Harlem's Wagner Houses stating that the complex had "become a battleground for gangbangers."[9] All of these articles center on the behavior of "violent" tenants and they promote a picture that blames public housing residents for why life in the projects is so dangerous and difficult.

Even in its COVID-19 coverage, the news media continued these fear-mongering narratives. A 2021 article in *The City* discusses increases in violent crimes that took place at NYCHA during the pandemic in 2020; highlighting statistics, the piece states: "shootings rose by 103%, from 155 to 314, while murders jumped by nearly 50%, from 47 to 70."[10] A local Bronx newspaper, the *Mott Haven Herald*, published an article, "South Bronx Gun Violence Spikes amid Pandemic," about the shooting of an eight-year-old girl in the borough's Patterson Houses.[11] A resident was quoted in the piece blaming the violence on boredom, stating "People have nothing to do."[12] A December 2020 CBS News article titled, "Staffer Delivering Food for Charity Shot on Upper West Side," discusses the shooting of two West Side Campaign Against Hunger workers who were shot at NYCHA's Amsterdam Houses while delivering food.[13] While I want to be careful not to minimize the issues of crime, violence, and mismanagement that have plagued some public housing developments, the media's razor-sharp focus on these narratives has left the general public believing that tenants live in constant fear for their lives and want nothing more than to escape the projects.

Those of us who call the projects home understand that the story is a lot more nuanced. Public housing complexes are communities with deep connections that have lasted generations. Like any close-knit community, we know our neighbors in the apartments next to us as well as on the floors and in buildings we share. We also look out for each other when in need, whether it's making a grocery store run for a neighbor, fixing a neighbor a plate of food when they need it, or donating clothes to a neighbor's child. It is this aspect of life in public housing that has been often overshadowed by accounts of despair and brutality. And these negative images feed attacks on the program. A. Scott Henderson posits in a 1995 essay, "'Tarred with the Exceptional Image': Public Housing and Popular Discourse, 1950–1990," that public housing's negative portrayal in the news media "likely encouraged opposition to continuing or expanding the program."[14] Expanding on Henderson's point, I would add that this warped portrait of public housing not only served to dissuade public support for continued investment in the program but also functioned as a tool to shift blame and responsibility for the program's shortcomings away from federal and local officials and onto residents.

May 25th, 2020

Our neighbor Ms. Diane has come over to catch my mother up on the latest community news and gossip, as she typically does. Ms. Diane informs my mother that the elevators in Building 6 are out of service, leaving elderly residents who depend on them to enter and leave stuck. Already vulnerable due to their age and socioeconomic position, our senior neighbors now had no way of traveling out of their building to purchase food and other essential items. Our tenant association president informed management about the issue and was told it may take a week to contract someone to fix the elevators. But there was no way we would wait a week, so we had an emergency tenant association meeting where we decided to have four young tenants get groceries and other essential items for senior residents who could not. We also decided that at least four of us would visit the management office every day until someone came to fix the elevators. For the next few days, I and three others collected lists of groceries and other items from five elderly residents, picked the items up from the supermarket, and delivered them to the tenants in Building 6. Four other tenants visited the management office during that period to file complaints about the broken elevators and inquire when they would be repaired. With persistent visits and threats to contact the media, by Friday management had contracted someone to repair the elevators. The lack of working elevators was a very serious maintenance concern that could have led to tenant deaths. NYCHA seemed ill-prepared or unwilling to deal with it in a timely manner; in the face of this, tenants stepped up to aid each other and pressure management. Stories like these have been absent from public dialogues concerning public housing's decades of woes.

Public housing has been afflicted by decades of neglect at both the state and federal levels. This neglect has routinely been placed at the feet of those of us who live there. The media pathologized the projects' mostly Black and POC poor and working-class residents, arguing that the dismal and deteriorating conditions within complexes have nothing to do with lack of maintenance and governmental underfunding and everything to do with tenants' behavior. Public housing residents have routinely been cast as the main culprits behind the depressing state of units: we are to blame, the story goes, because of our disregard for the place we live or because of our innate violence. But in reality, it has historically been tenants who have fought to improve conditions when governments and housing authorities have been unwilling or slow to do so. In the 1960s, Philadelphia public housing tenants, particularly Black women, according to historian Lisa Levenstein, "sought to claim ownership of their surroundings by decorating their apartments, maintaining public spaces, and forging relationships with neighbors."[15] This claiming of ownership over space also extended to the buildings themselves as tenants began demanding maintenance and infrastructural issues be handled and management resisted.[16] In the late 1960s, frustrated by a lack of repairs, maintenance, and a mouse and roach infestation, residents of Baltimore's O'Donnell Heights projects made complaints to management and the tenants' association to remedy these issues.[17] O'Donnell housing officials attempted to place blame for the problems facing the complex on tenants, and in response to this, the resident council sent a letter to officials that read in part: "Sure, some tenants do not take care of their homes and tear up the neighborhood. But are they the ones who made the electric wiring and the plumbing bad? Are they the ones who kept our buildings from being painted and let our porches fall apart?"[18] The 1970s saw the emergence of a tenant management movement as a response to what residents recognized as poor management by local housing authorities.[19] Numerous public housing tenants organized rent strikes across the country to get "local housing authorities to maintain complexes, replace broken building systems, and make repairs when necessary."[20] Tenants involved in this movement felt that management and maintenance began to decline once the projects' residents became predominantly Black. "But what happened was black people moved in and the services were gone," according to one resident.[21] As these historical examples show, public housing residents have been fighting for decades to deal with the debilitating state of project buildings despite efforts by housing authorities and news media to blame them for the conditions. This continues to be true for us public housing tenants; we have routinely had to pressure management to address maintenance and infrastructural concerns while simultaneously combatting narratives that seek to blame us for these problems.

Despite Albany Houses management's horrible handling of a maintenance concern during a global pandemic and other ongoing infrastructural issues, many of us who live in these projects are not seeking to escape; what we are seeking instead is for the government to care about public housing as much as we tenants do. In the media's coverage of the projects over the last fifty years, too often the voices of residents who have jettisoned all hope in the program have been spotlighted over those of us who recognize the importance of public housing to our lives and community. The media's focus on tenants who have given up on public housing has left the general public and elected officials believing that the program isn't worth investing in or preserving.

July 10th, 2020

Around this time of the year we would typically hold our annual summertime community event, Albany Day, but it has been canceled due to the pandemic. Albany Day is like a block party for our entire nine-building complex. It is a day when we celebrate the history of our community and acknowledge the individuals who have contributed to keeping our neighborhood thriving. We play music and dance, we barbecue on the lawns, kids play in the bouncy castles, and we laugh and relish each other's company. It is a cherished event that even former residents return to enjoy with friends or family members who still live here. Albany Day is one of the many examples of what makes the Albany Houses such a great community to live in.

My family and I have been residents of Albany Houses for over nineteen years; our neighbor Ms. Diane has lived here for twelve years; and another neighbor of ours, Ms. Christine, has called this complex home for eighteen years. A very important benefit we as public housing tenants have is the right to organize. Despite efforts by local housing authorities to thwart or obscure this right, HUD allows public housing tenants to organize and form tenant associations.[22] The federal government provides public housing authorities with funding that can be used to support residents councils and other tenant participatory activities.[23] Project residents cannot be evicted by housing authorities for complaining to media and government officials about conditions of the complex or for forming or joining tenant associations.[24] This makes public housing unique in that renters who live under private landlords don't have the same right and protection to organize, complain about conditions, and create tenant associations without fear of retribution. Public housing is also economically beneficial for its residents. A 2021 report from the Center on Budget and Policy Priorities shows that by lowering housing costs for its residents, public housing "leaves families with more resources for other expenses like food, health-related services, child care, and transportation."[25] The same report also states that public housing gives "older adults and people with disabilities the ability to remain in their home communities."[26] Public housing gives its low-income tenants financial stability that they would not have in the private housing market; given the outrageously expensive rents in New York City, it is likely that without public housing, most residents would have to leave the city.

The very financial security that living in the projects offers has resulted in the fostering of community bonds and ties between residents that have lasted generations. Too often, popular media narratives about public housing have pathologized long-term tenants as troubled, lazy, and dependent. The media doesn't show that residents are students, workers, organizers, community leaders, and advocates. The long-term stability provided by public housing has afforded many of my neighbors and me the opportunity to be upwardly mobile. For my neighbor Shannon, who used to sleep on a friend's couch with her daughter, the stability of living in public housing for five years allowed her to study for the MTA exam, pass it, and get a job that would have been a lot more difficult to obtain without a secure, supportive place to live. I am currently a doctoral student at the University of Massachusetts–Amherst, and I don't believe I would have gotten this far on my educational journey if it were not for the stability and community that public housing provided me. Relieved from the burden of having to stretch money to feed, clothe, and house myself, I was able to focus on my academic studies.

September 7th, 2020

I'm on Zoom for one of my graduate school seminars listening to my peers share their thoughts on the assigned book for the week. As I listen to each person's commentary, my mind becomes consumed with negative thoughts, and I begin comparing myself to my classmates:

"I wish I had made that point."

"They sound so much smarter than me."

"I could never articulate myself the way they do."

"Everyone probably thinks I'm dumb."

"I'm this struggling poor guy from the projects while they seem like they have everything together."

"They belong here more than I do."

"What am I doing here? I don't deserve to be here."

"I don't belong here."

"I don't belong . . ."

"I don't belong . . ."

"I don't belong . . ."

It is now a little over seven months into the pandemic and I have just begun my doctoral studies remotely. One thing I hadn't anticipated at the start of this pandemic was the impact it would have on me mentally and emotionally. I was depressed and anxious, but I didn't realize it until I was in the midst of my graduate classes. Learning for me has always been a communal experience; I would not have gotten through my undergraduate studies without the community bonds that I was able to foster inside and outside the classroom. But the pandemic, when all classes were on Zoom, made connecting with my doctoral program peers more difficult. The isolation I was already feeling from the impact of the pandemic on my neighborhood, coupled with being isolated from my class peers, led me to feel depressed and anxious. The depression and anxiety affected two extremely important skills needed to complete graduate school: reading and writing. I found it very difficult to finish assigned books because I lacked the motivation or will to do so. Completing written assignments was even harder because I would become crippled with anxiety and negative thoughts to the point where I couldn't continue writing. Graduate school already comes with its set of mentally and emotionally taxing experiences (many students have to navigate imposter syndrome), but the pandemic exacerbated them. And the community that students would typically lean on to help mitigate these challenges was disrupted by the pandemic.

My mental and emotional state had me using the very thing—my status as a public housing resident—that helped me get into graduate school as a weapon to question my placement in the program. Not only did public housing provide a stable environment for me to be able to pursue a college education, but it is also at the center of my scholarly research interests. Yet here I was using my background as a public housing tenant to question whether I deserved or belonged in grad school.

I realized I had internalized many of the racist and anti-poor and working-class sentiments that have been spewed about my community. The same rhetoric that told us we weren't worthy or deserving I was regurgitating back onto myself. People from subjugated communities like mine, even those of us who are relatively conscious, often internalize the rhetoric of the dominant class. The pressures of graduate school, along with the stress of the pandemic, had me questioning myself and my capabilities. Even the completion of this piece was impacted by my mental health condition. I would eventually seek aid from the campus counselor that my program referred me to but even this felt like little help to me because it was virtual. I longed for a return to some type of normalcy. I longed for the ability to build and foster community with my peers on campus in person. I longed for the return of my community at Albany Houses where beneath the avalanche of governmental underfunding and neglect and media narratives of pathology lies a people who look out for and take care of one another.

Being raised in a neglected and crumbling public housing complex, I grew to profoundly appreciate the importance of community. I cherish and value my community not just because of the memories we build in leisure, but also because when NYCHA and state and federal government officials fall short of keeping our community safe and secure, it has been my neighbors who have continually stepped up to meet the challenge. Due to the preexisting condition of neglect and dilapidation, when the pandemic hit, we already had years of experience organizing to aid each other in times of need. Despite decades of rhetoric from the media and elected officials tethering the project's shortcomings to the behavior of its tenants, residents of Albany Houses have shown us that the narrative is the other way around. Public housing residents aren't the cause behind the program's woes, we are the catalyst behind the push to remedy issues. The pandemic has led to a critical focus on how NYCHA is run, with many news articles criticizing the housing authority for the poor state of its buildings and the increased risk it put tenants in during the pandemic. While I'm certainly not opposed to criticisms of NYCHA's deteriorating infrastructure—residents have been making similar complaints for years—I don't believe the media's critiques are rooted in wanting to preserve public housing, but are instead part of the effort to privatize the program. Since 2016, through their Permanent Affordability Commitment Together (PACT) program, NYCHA began leasing their public housing properties to private companies in exchange for funding to deal with maintenance and infrastructural issues.[27] PACT is New York City's version of the federal Rental Assistance Demonstration (RAD) program which claims to be aimed at preserving public housing, but remedies the project's lack of money by allowing local housing authorities to seek outside funding sources.[28] The Manhattanville Houses,

Audubon Houses, Williamsburg Houses, and Murphy Houses are just a few of the NYCHA developments that were leased to private companies under PACT.[29] Through PACT, these developments are no longer run by NYCHA which means maintenance of the buildings, as well as rent and leases, are the responsibility of the private company.[30] Investigations have already revealed that Ocean Bay Houses, the first NYCHA development converted via PACT, had higher rates of eviction following the conversion than under NYCHA management.[31] The media's focus on stories of NYCHA's disastrous mismanagement, in the absence of a call to preserve government-run and operated public housing, only aids in privatization efforts like PACT.

What this pandemic has shown is the vital importance of public housing as a tool to meet the housing needs of the nation's most economically vulnerable citizens. A study by the Community Service Society of New York found that during the pandemic Asian, Black, and Latinx NYC tenants were three to four times more likely than white tenants to have fallen behind on rent payments.[32] This same study also found that Asian, Black, and Latinx tenants were two to three times more likely than whites to be unsure they could pay next month's rent.[33] Following the January 2022 lifting of New York State's rent moratorium, landlords had made over 43,000 eviction filings.[34] *Gothamist* published data from the New York City Department of Investigation that showed a steady increase in evictions after the end of the rent moratorium, with the highest number of evictions taking place in November of 2022.[35] New York's pandemic-era moratorium on evictions was crucial, but only provided a band-aid solution to the much larger problem: the lack of affordable housing. The *New York Times* published an article citing a study that showed that half of the city's residents could not afford to "comfortably pay rent, access sufficient food and basic health care, or get around."[36] Despite the growing unaffordability of New York City housing for poor and working-class people, officials don't seem to have an adequate solution to this issue.

Public housing could have prevented this crisis and solved it, yet the media and elected officials continue to be disinterested in putting it forward as a solution due to the years of scrutiny it has received. Public housing remains the only truly affordable housing option for the city's most economically disadvantaged residents. Only through reinvesting in the program at both the state and federal level, so that old buildings are revitalized and new ones can be constructed, will this affordable housing crisis end. In order for a national reinvestment in the program to occur, the image of public housing needs to be rehabbed. While scholars have been doing the work of challenging and demystifying myths about the projects, this work needs to be directed and facilitated by public housing residents. It has been residents of communities like Albany Houses who have consistently led the fight to make public housing safe, comfortable, and livable even when local and federal officials failed to do so. News media rhetoric paints tenants as the violent and deviant culprits behind public housing's problems. But, in reality we are victims of governmental neglect and underfunding who have always had to rely on each other.

CHAPTER 14

COVID-19: Mortality by Zip Code

Marsha Decatus

"Tell me where you live, and I'll tell you about your health."

With sobering sincerity, my Introduction to Public Health professor spoke these words.

I was a senior.

And an exhausted biology major.

I never paused to consider the social determinants of health. As my professor took the semester to explain the meaning behind his words, I listened.

Nine months into the pandemic, I heard his voice again as I read an Association of American Medical Colleges (AAMC) article stating "COVID-19 mortality is six times higher in areas that are predominately non-white as compared to areas that are predominately white." I grew tired of articles noting "hypertension, obesity, and diabetes" and blaming living environments "marked by poverty, high housing density, and high crime rates" for the higher mortality rates plaguing communities of color.[1] Reporting COVID-19 risk factors without historical context felt incomplete and ignored the structural forces driving health inequity. Still, I scoured the article for a challenge to the narrative that COVID-19 mortality was an inevitable consequence of Black and Brown life.

I found relief as the AAMC article linked COVID-19 mortality to a long history of racial segregation in the United States. Yet, public health experts emphasized only preventive measures to preserve life. How could the most vulnerable communities effectively practice social distancing when their physical environment precluded this possibility? Systemic disinvestment in areas such as Boston, New York, Philadelphia, and Washington, DC left communities of color under-resourced without adequate personal protective equipment. As social distancing and diligent mask use were touted as life-saving remedies, I considered how different my life might have been had I called somewhere else home.

I lived my formative years at 440 Lenox Road—an East Flatbush apartment building across from SUNY Downstate Medical Center. I remembered this Brooklyn two-bedroom apartment for its living room the most—a space where I spent most of my time. The creaky floors alerted my mother each time I attempted to watch *Sailor Moon* before school and informed my father of my surprise attacks whenever he converted the living room to his personal study. Beyond our quiet walls, I lived for my neighborhood's culture and activity. There was a collective hustle among East Flatbush residents. Drivers expertly coordinated their arrivals and departures to snag available parking spots once alternate side parking restrictions ended. Our local grocery stores supplied fresh herbs and spices for our homemade "epis" marinade and offered ripe green plantains to accompany our savory proteins. Every day, I watched as Black and Brown faces in white coats scurried into the nearby hospital to tend to their patients. On any given day, my favorite security guard sang "Hi Marsha!" in his West Indian accent when I entered the apartment building.

I walked ten minutes to my elementary school, St. Catherine of Genoa, where faculty and staff poured into my academic and personal success. I discovered my singing ability in their afterschool program and grew fond of the counselors who encouraged my individuality when I wanted to conform. Twice a week, my parents and I took a fifteen-minute drive to Bonnii's Dance Showcase where I cultivated my love for dance. As an eight-year-old girl, surrounded by family, culture, and the opportunity to realize my potential, I felt I had all I needed.

In 1998, I learned a different style of Brooklyn-living when my parents and I moved twenty minutes south to Old Mill Basin. As we drove to our new home in Brooklyn's eighteenth district, Flatlands/Canarsie, I immediately noticed the tree-lined streets, Italian bakeries and specialty grocery stores, and multiple supermarkets.[2] Located on a peaceful corner plot, this single-family home had more space than I had grown accustomed to. The finished basement became my playroom, where I escaped my mother's gaze as I watched my cartoons. I no longer interrupted my father as he worked; the smallest bedroom became his home office. Our new home had a garage, though I often questioned if we needed it: there was always a lengthy parking spot in front of the house. I walked five minutes to my new elementary school, Mary, Queen of Heaven School, one block away from our new home. It took fifteen minutes to walk to The Dance Spot—one of four dance schools in the area. I chose between two libraries when exploring new genres and frequented Marine Park for recreation with friends.

While I enjoyed Old Mill Basin for its conveniences and amenities, I missed how "at-home" I felt in our previous East Flatbush abode. The new grocery stores, while plentiful, rarely shelved our Haitian staples. If we did find ripe plantains and fresh cloves, they were sold at a higher price. I turned to neighboring communities, Canarsie and Flatbush, for hair health and styling needs as the Old Mill Basin pharmacies and salons could not tend to my kinky tresses. As I traveled outside of my neighborhood for products that served my truest self, I wondered why my cultural identity seemed at odds with my new neighborhood's resources. Just like the electrical hum of fluorescent lights you cannot unhear after someone calls your attention to them, I could not shake this feeling as I continued my secondary schooling further west, in Bay Ridge.

Fontbonne Hall Academy was unlike any high school I had seen on my favorite sitcoms *Family Matters* or *Saved by the Bell*. Lauded for its extensive alumni network, professional status-holding parents, and white gown graduations, Fontbonne boasted academic rigor with finishing school touches. Were it not for Fontbonne's cobalt blue emblem with embossed gold lettering, I would not know this converted mansion was actually a school. There was no squat, rectangular building with tile-floored classrooms or a gymnasium that doubled as the site for homecoming dances or proms. Instead, a black cast iron gate surrounded several two- and three-story buildings and adjoining courtyard to create a campus suitable for five hundred young women. Still, Fontbonne's presence extended beyond those gates. The annual "Walk-a-thon" event took place along the neighboring walkway, Shore Parkway. In warmer months, we strode across the street to Shore Road Park to practice our tennis swings for physical education. During the Senior Year Fashion Show fundraiser, I modeled an elegant, bespoke gown from a boutique two blocks away, on Third Avenue.

As I immersed myself in Fontbonne's traditions, I took stock of my Bay Ridge surroundings: the only source of noise came from the laughter of my fellow "Bonnies"; the perfectly manicured lawns that appeared green all year long; the graceful six-story apartment buildings that overlooked the Narrows, a tidal strait separating Brooklyn and Staten Island; and the almost exclusively white residents that inhabited the area.[3] Aside from the patrons on Eighty-Sixth Street, the neighborhood's shopping and transportation hub, and the few fellow "Bonnies" of color, I rarely saw people who looked like me. Nearly fifteen years later, not much has changed. I did not know then that I had witnessed the vestiges of housing policies established ninety years prior.

During the Great Depression, many Americans struggled to make their mortgage payments and eventually lost their homes. In response, the federal government established the Home Owners' Loan Corporation (HOLC), which refinanced urban mortgages in danger of default and granted low-interest loans to borrowers who lost their homes through foreclosure.[4] To determine relief recipients, the HOLC appraised each community for its lending desirability according to ethnic composition, housing quality, and potential for business growth. Using these criteria, the organization developed a residential security map for banks to use categorized into four distinct grades, lettered "A" through "D."[5]

Zones with the two highest grades, A and B, received the most lending support. Areas coded A were described as "best" and displayed in green. These sections had recent home improvements, an upper-middle-class population, and potential for future business development. B-graded communities were highlighted in blue. Though "still desirable" for lending, for their well-maintained homes, proximity to parks, and professional status-holding residents, these districts were "completely developed" and had "reached their peak" in terms of business development. C-labeled communities were considered "definitely declining" and usually had a high percentage of racial and ethnic minority residents. Neighborhoods graded C were marked in yellow for their "disagreeable" populations, poor maintenance of homes, or obsolete housing.[6]

The final set of communities were graded D and displayed in red. D-labeled communities were deemed "hazardous" for lending. Marked by poverty, dilapidated homes, and an "infiltration of Negroes," defined as more than 5% Black residency, areas coded D proved unfit for mortgage investment. As Black communities were coded red and denied loans for their "heavy financial risk," the discriminatory lending practice—redlining—had officially made its debut.[7]

The HOLC granted the site of my first East Flatbush apartment a B-. During the 1930s, the area, then labeled by the HOLC as Flatbush (Holy Cross) Brooklyn for its proximity to Holy Cross Cemetery, was home to skilled laborers of Jewish, Irish, and Italian heritage. The area boasted recent construction, "good transportation," and numerous playgrounds, but its two-fare zoning, proximity to then named Brooklyn State Hospital for the "mentally defi-cient" (now Kingsboro Psychiatric Center), and ethnic mixture lowered the community desirability of East Flatbush. The HOLC gave my current home, Old Mill Basin, and its surrounding communities a C. Then categorized as Flatlands, Brooklyn, the area experienced public improvements, such as the Brooklyn-Queens Circumferential Parkway, which enabled vehicles to avoid Brooklyn's congestion and connected to the Bronx, Westchester, and New England. Flatlands' bays fed into the Atlantic Ocean. The residents, primarily city employees, took pride in home ownership. While unpaved streets, vacant areas, and proximity to dumps lowered the neighborhood's value, the Irish and British inhabitants buoyed the community's desirability. Finally, twenty minutes west, a booming business site bordering the Narrows of New York Harbor received the HOLC's highest evaluation. The area boasted a land-scaped Shore Road Drive and reasonable distance from noise and heavy traf-fic. Business executives and professionals of Irish and British origin further increased the HOLC score. The single "A" rating in all of Brooklyn, located in the Southwest corner of Bay Ridge, would become home to my Alma Mater, Fontbonne Hall Academy. Just like that, redlining had taught me a lesson in American values. While neighborhood amenities piqued investment inter-ests, desirable demographics drove economic investment.[8]

As banks adopted the HOLC's residential security maps to determine which neighborhoods were safe (or conversely, hazardous) for lending, investment (and conversely, disinvestment) spread throughout Brooklyn. The HOLC's greatest influence, however, was found in the underwriting practices of the Federal Housing Administration (FHA)—a government agency whose function was to insure mortgages. As the FHA guaranteed 90% of the prop-erty value, thereby adequately securing housing loans, the federal govern-ment eliminated the risk to banks and lowered the interest rates charged to borrowers. FHA provisions, coupled with new construction techniques, were responsible for the housing boom nationwide, and more significantly, the exodus of middle-class, white residents from cities to suburbs.[9]

The FHA's housing stipulations and heavy reliance on "unbiased" property appraisals were yet another systemic barrier for people of color. Minimum standards for lot size and setbacks favored the construction of single-family homes and excluded attached (read: Black) inner-city dwell-ings from eligibility. For middle-class, white Brooklynites, the FHA require-ments catalyzed the abandonment of Northern and Central Brooklyn districts in exchange for newly attractive areas along Brooklyn's Southern periphery. Once white residents settled into their new communities, they worked diligently to maintain neighborhood homogeneity to protect their new investment. For Black Brooklynites, however, the discriminatory lending practices and white flight forced African American and Caribbean residents into North Brooklyn. As a result, Brooklyn's northern sections were underdeveloped and drained of municipal resources to meet the growing demands of South Brooklyn. By the 1960s, Brooklyn's previously most desirable neighborhoods had turned into slums, but the resulting vacancies created an opportunity for home ownership. Black Brooklynites across the socioeconomic strata moved to northern and central Brooklyn in droves, finding housing in Prospect Heights, Clinton Hill, Bedford-Stuyvesant, Crown Heights, Brownsville, East New York, Flatbush, and East Flatbush. Altogether, the communities became Black Brooklyn—the largest contiguous Black area of New York City.[10]

Fort Greene, Brooklyn highlights the demographic shift. In 1960, an estimated sixteen thousand white residents and fourteen thousand Black residents lived in the area. However, by 1970, the Black population increased to eighteen thousand while the white population plummeted to a mere seven thousand residents. As the face of Fort Greene shifted from white to Black, the priorities of the Black working class influenced the neighborhood's culture. Shaped by the Black Freedom Movement, Fort Greene's political, religious, and community organizations challenged housing discrimination, boycotted local businesses that refused to hire minorities, and demanded an end to public school segregation and overcrowding. When the Black middle class arrived in the 1980's, however, their concept of community control was less radical. While Black middle-class residents valued decent housing and adequate schools, they did not necessarily support public housing, working-class establishments, or radical political ideas. Still, the middle-class newcomers took over civic associations, church groups, block associations, and political organizations to address Fort Greene's challenges, often considering the future of their working-class neighbors. Yet the Black working-class residents felt the middle-class interventions were paternalistic and eventually resented their middle-class neighbors. Despite this dissonance, Black Brooklynites had a place they could call "their own." By the 1990s, Black Brooklyn was recognized as the "the New Black Mecca"; Fort Greene and the adjacent neighborhood, Clinton Hill, were epicenters of a national Black Renaissance.

Despite the strides Black Brooklyn made in Black art and fashion, business, and entrepreneurship, Black Brooklynites could not contend with the legacy of federal disinvestment. The remnants of the crack epidemic still littered "the New Black Mecca" as crack addicts took up residence on Fort Greene corners. Redlining had effectively established non-white Brooklyn communities and primed them for disproportionately poor health outcomes.[11]

Forty years later, COVID-19 mortality rates follow these same racialized, residential patterns. In 2019, there were approximately 136,009 residents living in my first childhood neighborhood East Flatbush, Brooklyn. The demographics are as follows: 85.8% identified as Black, 7.6% as Hispanic, 2.3% as Asian, and 2.5% as white. Of the 21,179 residents diagnosed with COVID-19 as of 2022, 476 died of the disease. My current home in Old Mill Basin, by comparison, had a larger population—196,895 residents—of which 62.5% identified as Black, 9.1% as Hispanic, 5.4% as Asian and 21.4% as white. While 27,822 of these Flatlands/Canarsie residents contracted COVID-19 (that is 6,643 more than East Flatbush's incidence), 441 residents (35 fewer than East Flatbush) died from the disease.[12]

Finally, Bay Ridge/Dyker Heights, home to my alma mater, had an estimated resident population of 121,925, of which 2.1% identified as Black, 17.8% as Hispanic, 23.6% as Asian, and 53.6% as white. Of the 22,810 total incident cases, 290 residents died from COVID-19. As expected, Bay Ridge, the only area in all of Brooklyn to have received an HOLC "A" rating, demonstrated the lowest mortality rate of the three communities. However, the mortality rate of my current neighborhood, Old Mill Basin experienced 35 *fewer* deaths than East Flatbush despite receiving the worst HOLC rating of the three sections in 1933.[13]

Here lies the crux of the opening article I cited: neighborhood racial composition predicts health outcomes. Structural racism clusters Black and Brown communities into socioeconomic disadvantage, which in turn predisposes non-white residents to poorer health. Often, such outcomes are unavoidable, despite individual, health-conscious efforts. Therefore, systemic disinvestment, established through the HOLC's discriminatory grading system, drives health inequity. The relationship between systemic neglect (or conversely, investment) and health is further elucidated as previous patterns of out-migration during the 1960s reversed in the 1990s. As renewed interest in urban centers grew across the nation, Brooklyn's previously abandoned northern and central sections became increasingly attractive for their proximity to Manhattan, robust transportation services, historic brownstones, and luxury condominium investment opportunities. Additionally, Rudolph Giuliani, New York City's mayor from 1994 to 2001, "cleaned up the city" to make affluent residents and visitors comfortable in NYC's urban environments. New York City revitalization ensued. As NYC's administration promoted its safer and "cleaner" cities, white residents poured into Black Brooklyn's neighborhoods. The population influx to the borough, associated with neighborhood revitalization, is known as the back-to-the-city phenomenon. As northern and central Brooklyn's neighborhood population became whiter, conditions improved, and so did its residents' health outcomes.[14]

The celebrated Black Brooklyn neighborhood of Bedford-Stuyvesant, affectionately known as Bed-Stuy, showcases the influence of the back-to-the-city movement on health. In two short decades, Bed-Stuy experienced a nearly fifteenfold increase in white residency, a factor I use to measure the movement's increasing popularity. In 2000, Bedford-Stuyvesant had a resident population that was 74.9% Black, 19.0% Hispanic, 2.4% white, and 0.8% Asian. By 2019, Bed-Stuy's diversity increased as the residents identified as 45.6% Black, 19.5% Hispanic, 29.4% white, and 3.0% Asian. During this time, Bed-Stuy experienced notable changes in its physical and economic environment. Air quality improved. In 2009, the average fine particulate matter level—the burden of harmful particles emitted by combustion sources—was 10.75. By 2020, Bed-Stuy's average fine particulate matter level decreased to 6.2. The fresher air reduced the likelihood of Bed-Stuy residents contracting respiratory disease. Additionally, in 2016, Bed-Stuy contained fifty-seven bodegas for every one supermarket. In just four years, the number decreased to eighteen bodegas—nearly one-third of the original statistic. The improvement came at a cost, however. While the decrease in bodegas created a healthier food environment for Bed-Stuy residents, the residual income needed to sustain a healthier diet also increased. According to a Harvard study, a day's worth of the healthiest diet pattern costs about $1.50 more per day than the least healthy ones. Over the course of a year, that is an additional $550 for an individual to eat healthier.[15] Fortunately, Bed-Stuy experienced a significant increase in income. In 2000, the median household income was $37,560. By 2019, the median income had increased to $64,300. While Bed-Stuy's median was lower than the citywide median of $72,930, the increased income allowed Bedford-Stuyvesant residents to afford healthier choices. For instance, sugary drink consumption decreased among adults. In 2008, 46.3% of adults consumed at least one sugary drink per day in Bed-Stuy. By 2020, adult sugar drink consumption decreased to 27.2%.[16]

The aforementioned enhancements allowed Bed-Stuy residents better living conditions, which in turn supported improved health outcomes. Since heightened particulate matter levels triggered asthma, the improved air quality decreased asthma cases—the leading cause of emergency room visits, hospitalizations, and missed school days in New York City's poorest neighborhoods. In 2005, the number of emergency room asthma cases for patients aged five to seventeen in Bed-Stuy was 1,785; by 2018, the ER cases decreased to 1,537. Most significant, however, was Bed-Stuy's decline in infant mortality—death among children before age one. While infant mortality had improved boroughwide, Bed-Stuy's cases were among the highest. In 1998, Bed-Stuy had sixty-three infant mortality cases—one-fourth of Brooklyn's infant deaths. Fifteen years later, as mass in-migration spurred neighborhood investment, Bedford-Stuyvesant's infant mortality decreased to twenty-seven cases—nearly one-fifth of Brooklyn's infant mortality. In 1957, when 86% of all Black Brooklynites lived in Bedford-Stuyvesant, the infant mortality rate was *one-third higher* than Brooklyn's borough-wide rate. Bed-Stuy experienced remarkable changes in infant mortality in just five short decades; community revitalization was the catalyst. As Bed-Stuy's living environment and health outcomes improved, its revitalized sections were better equipped to grapple with COVID-19.[17]

Sections of Bed-Stuy experienced varying degrees of COVID-19 mortality. Bedford-Stuyvesant includes four zip codes—11205, 11216, 11221, and 11233; each zip code includes a neighboring community with different percentages of white residency. Again, I use the demographic shift within Bed-Stuy's neighboring communities to showcase neighborhood revitalization and highlight the influence such revitalization has on Bed-Stuy's COVID-19 mortality rates. Zip code 11205 (Fort Greene/Clinton Hill to the West) in 2000 had an estimated white population that was 31.1%; but in 2019, white residents made up 52.1% of Fort Greene/Clinton Hill's population. Similarly, 11216, which includes Crown Heights West located south of Bed-Stuy, experienced an in-migration of white residents. In 2000, white residency was 7.4%; nineteen years later, white residency increased to four times the statistic, 30.8%. In zip codes 11205 and 11216, where white residency increased considerably, the COVID-19 death rate as of November 10, 2022, was 264.71 and 348.38 per 100,000, respectively—both lower than Brooklyn's borough-wide COVID-19 mortality rate, 417.13 per 100,000.

The mortality rates of the remaining zip codes—11221 and 11233—were 446.95 and 503.21 per 100,000, respectively, as of November 10, 2022. These zip codes have greater COVID-19 mortality rates than Brooklyn's aforesaid borough-wide rate. Zip code 11221 includes Bushwick, just east of Bed-Stuy. Its white residency was 3.1% in 2000; by 2019, Bushwick's white residency increased sevenfold, to 20.6%. Zip code 11233, which includes Brownsville just South of Bed-Stuy, is an interesting case. While the white resident population increased from 0.7% in 2000 to 3.8% in 2019, Brownsville's white residency is the lowest of all Bed-Stuy's zip codes. As of 2019, the race and ethnicity profile of Brownsville's remaining residents is 0.9% Asian, 68.4% Black, and 25.6% Hispanic. As of late 2022, Brownsville's other zip code, 11212, suffered Brooklyn's second-highest COVID-19 mortality rate—755.74 per 100,000. Like Bed-Stuy, Brownsville was a former Black Brooklyn neighborhood, but Brownsville has not experienced the same level of revitalization as Bedford-Stuyvesant's other sections. Therefore, COVID-19 mortality, like other health outcomes, reflects the patterns of disinvestment consistently seen in predominantly Black and Brown neighborhoods.[18]

What do the disproportionate rates of COVID-19 mortality among Black and Brown communities demonstrate? Historically, federal institutions, such as the HOLC and FHA, valued whiteness. Accordingly, private and public entities followed suit. Gentrification then changed parts of the city, and investment followed white migration. The consequences of such a value system led to greater investment in white neighborhoods than in non-white neighborhoods; greater employment opportunities, cleaner air, and better-quality food for white residents than non-white residents; and by extension, better health outcomes for white people than their non-white peers. COVID-19 is no exception. No amount of masking and assiduous hand washing could spare Black and Brown communities from the vestiges of structural racism. Even more painful than the countless Black and Brown lives lost to the disease? In this country, with our history, disproportionate COVID-19 mortality rates remain endemic among communities of color. I now understand why my professor spoke earnestly as he asserted the link between one's zip code and health. As I analyzed Brooklyn's COVID-19 mortality rates, his words rang true.

CHAPTER 15

We See from Where We Stand: COVID-19 and the Shape of Us

Donna-Lee Granville

"We shape our society, and our society shapes us." I've probably uttered a version of this statement a hundred times each semester for at least the last five years. This dialectical relationship expresses what sociologists focus on—the link between *structure*, or the rules and systems that organize and distribute resources differentially, and *agency*, the power and free will of individuals. Usually, it comes after we've spent an entire class session pretending that we are all in a bathroom together. The urinal game we play usually goes like this:[1]

In the center of the classroom are four empty chairs. I ask for five student volunteers and tell them that they are simply to pretend that we've all been transported to a public bathroom where the chairs are stalls, and they decide how they will use the bathroom based on conditions that I manipulate. The first student typically has it the easiest. Being careful to note where the entrance to the bathroom is, I ask them to share what stall they would choose and ask their classmates to share if they agree or disagree with the choice. As each student gets a chance to choose their stall, the conditions change. What stall would you choose if they are all full or only two of the four are working? Would you use this bathroom if the stalls had no doors? How would your choices change if this was a co-ed bathroom?

Inevitably, in classes as varied as Introduction to Sociology, Race and Ethnicity, and the Sociology of Hip Hop, students quickly arrive at similar conclusions. The bathroom is an example of how our society has decided to respond to a specific issue; the fact that humans need to relieve themselves outside of their own homes. How our stalls are organized—including the oft-lamented space between stalls—and the rules of behavior that govern our bathroom use reflect the structure and culture of the society we live in. In our discussions after this activity, students note how invisible ideas of gender, stigma, shame, and deviance influence their behavior toward the norm. They also notice how the physical arrangement of the bathroom—whether a single bathroom or one with multiple stalls, or if it is accessible for those living with disabilities—changes its efficiency despite its necessity.

An essential part of what I do as a sociology professor is to show students how choices like the ones they make in a bathroom are both facilitated and inhibited by the structure of the society they live in. At its core, my job is to awaken my students' *sociological imagination*. When sociologists use this term, we are referring to a way of seeing and understanding the world that makes us aware that what we experience and participate in is the result of what we think and do as individuals and groups with different levels of power. As the world shifted into crisis mode due to the COVID-19 pandemic, I found myself revisiting these ideas with renewed interest. What good is a sociological imagination in these times if it merely reveals the structures that enclose us and not the path to our liberation as well?

First articulated by C. Wright Mills in 1959, the sociological imagination encourages us to connect individual and group patterns to the culture, institutions, and rules that govern a specific society. Mills was concerned about people finding themselves in a trap, unable to understand how their personal issues were related to the structural forces that govern the society they live in. For Mills, the sociological imagination was the ideal remedy. An active sociological imagination doesn't just reveal the material conditions of our existence. It questions why things are the way they are and critiques whether the structures and institutions that give shape to our lives make sense for our evolving realities. Where common sense, rumors, and gossip can confound, the gift of a sociological imagination is a necessary lucidity about the dynamics of the world we live in. It grants the ability to recognize how events taking place in our world around us influence our options and choices. Thinking sociologically invites us to see and interrogate our lived experiences as tangible reminders that "neither the life of an individual nor the history of a society can be understood without understanding both."[2]

The narratives in *Until We're Seen* are proof that the sociological imagination has not lost its utility. In each chapter of this book, the scenes, settings, main actors, and supporting players that make cameos throughout these stories are artful demonstrations of how to consider the consequences of our history and biography in the present moment. In this section, the narrations of Dominick Braswell, Marsha Decatus, Areeba Zanub, and Anthony Almojera boldly address some of the most pressing public issues of this time: housing insecurity, residential segregation, an inefficient health care system, and inadequate mental health services. Their stories point to the institutions, or conventional and accepted ways of accomplishing necessary societal tasks, that lump and split us into groups that determine our access to resources needed for our survival. The valued, the undervalued, and the devalued; the essential and non-essential; the privileged and the "truly disadvantaged." By telling their stories these student ethnographers are engaging in a necessary form of activism: the work of raising our consciousness. In doing so, their narratives accentuate the sociological truth that "where we stand determines what we're able to see."[3]

Dominick's and Anthony's standpoints acknowledge the "inescapable web of mutuality" that makes us interdependent whether we like it or not. Their narratives amplify how our choices and personal sacrifices configure communities that offer temporary and incomplete solutions to collective problems. In his piece, Dominick addresses the legacy of government neglect and disinvestment in New York City public housing. He is careful to note the roles played by the media and policy makers, who perpetuate controlling images that further pathologize those who reside there—often poor people of color and other marginalized groups. Taking matters into their own hands, these already vulnerable people attempted to fill in the gaps that widened during COVID-19. Dominick details the network of neighbors—young, old, and in between—who came together to address the various issues that the pandemic compounded. As he writes about how this group of tenants strategized to deal with a broken elevator, he illustrates how "communities sustain life."[4] At the same time, they shouldn't have to. Dominick rightfully critiques NYCHA for its willful ignorance of tenant rights and their issues and paints a vivid picture of community life that champions their humanity. His description of the empty community center and playground, Ms. Angela's absence and the card game that isn't taking place in the lobby explain how COVID-19 disrupted community life. Dominick's piece counters many of the tropes that plague our understanding of public housing and prevent us from seeing how it should and could be a vehicle for social mobility. That it isn't is related to who it benefits and the devaluation of those who need it most.

Anthony Almojera's essay does the same work for health care. He begins with a jarring memory of having to tell a mother that she would outlive her son. As a diabetic, her son died because of the consequences of rationing the insulin his body needed to survive. As Anthony sees it, "The fact that in the world's richest country scenes like this take place daily and are exacerbated by the COVID-19 pandemic is a stain on our American souls." He's right. Anthony wastes no time placing much deserved blame on our failure to institute meaningful health care reform that affords us all access to the care we need. Though quantifying the impact of COVID-19 through numbers and statistics has its value, these statistics are an abstraction of the real lives cut short and the impact of losing a loved one on the living. Anthony also gives voice and imagery to the fear and overwhelming conditions the city's 911 system endured. While I can viscerally recall the anxiety I heard every time an ambulance turned on its siren, I seldom thought about the burden borne by EMS workers tasked with being first responders. While we clapped for nurses and doctors, how often did we thank EMS personnel for their personal commitments to a traumatic job?

Anthony's piece was striking for what it revealed about the untenable working conditions faced by the small EMS community that the city relies on for a myriad of emergencies. The irony that EMTs get only twelve days of sick leave while being asked to take care of sick people is a cruel example of exploitation and alienation. EMTs being forced to start GoFundMe websites to meet their health care costs is akin to the mobilizing that Dominick and the other tenants did to get their broken elevator fixed. Though Anthony and Dominick write about different institutions, a crucial thread connects them. When our institutions fail us, our individual and collective response is to close the gap ourselves to meet our immediate needs. This ensures that our very resilience can be weaponized against us and solutions to our suffering can be repackaged as commodities to soothe us. It goes against the empowerment Mills envisioned as the result of sociological thinking. Yet, while Mills lamented the "pervasive transformation" that "ordinary men"[5] internally experience because of the societies they live in, he stops short of interrogating how the sociocultural, political, and economic conditions we find ourselves in obscure our vision, leaving us struggling to imagine other possibilities to the structural forces that determine our life chances.

Marsha's and Areeba's essays are made possible by their ability to straddle this two-ness and develop a second sight about their lived experiences and social locations as members of marginalized communities. Yet they also demonstrate the ease with which resilience becomes an insufficient stand-in for resistance and revolution. For Areeba, community is centered in her experience as a Pakistani immigrant to New York. In Marsha's narrative, community refers to Brooklyn's neighborhoods and the life chances you are afforded—or not—based on where you live. Their stories are also about how the past is always present even if we choose to ignore it.

Areeba opens her essay with a poetic reflection on her mental health journey that begins with fainting spells in her adolescence and teen years. Her mental health declined during the pandemic, and her struggles to manage her anxiety were shared by countless others, including me. What at first seems to be a story about how cultural histories shape our approaches to compassion and care soon becomes a deeper meditation on how individuals bear the burden of community trauma and on the transmission of trauma across cleavages of power in the doctor's office or in a family. When Areeba writes that "generational trauma is not just the infliction of trauma but also the denial of trauma," those words are derived from her experiences within a Pakistani community that she critiques but that she also loves and protects. Seeing beyond the present to find the legacy of a traumatic past and beyond her own mental health to the wellness of her community is a quintessential example of the interplay of history and biography.

Where Areeba centers her experience to tell her story, Marsha Decatus probes the data about COVID-19's disparate racial impact through a detailed exploration of Brooklyn's residential history. A Brooklyn native, Marsha considers "how differently my life might have been had I called somewhere else home." Her lived experiences in East Flatbush, Mill Basin, and Bay Ridge serve as an initiation to her personal neighborhood history and to her standpoint. As she traverses these neighborhoods, she notes the changes. Tree-lined streets with ample parking space. No Haitian food items in the grocery store. Salons unable to cater to kinky hair. Unsatisfied with the lack of context provided to explain why Black and brown Brooklynites had higher numbers of COVID-19 infection and mortality, Marsha weaves together an impressive amount of data to make the connection transparent for us. What she finds is that COVID-19 statistics are connected to racial residential segregation and housing policies that span almost a century. When whites settle in a Brooklyn neighborhood, the economic revitalization that occurs encourages the addition of resources that translate to better health outcomes—not just COVID-19. The most compelling data case is Bed-Stuy. Using data on income, racial demographics, infant mortality, and air quality, Marsha shows how Bed-Stuy's health outcomes improved as the neighborhood became less Black, more middle class, and more white. In neighborhoods like Browns-ville, once predominantly Black, a much smaller influx of whites has not yet inspired as much economic revitalization. A fact that Marsha shows is reflected in Brownsville reporting the second-highest COVID-19 mortality rate in Brooklyn.

The autoethnographies shared in this section of *Until We're Seen* tell stories about people making a living amid state neglect in health care and housing, institutional racism, oppression, redlining and gentrification, white supremacy, anti-Blackness, and racial capitalism, to name a few structural forces of significance. These brilliant essays attest to the amount of work it takes to see ourselves and our position in the world when structures maintain their power precisely because of the illusions and limitations they naturalize in our lives. Areeba mined her personal history to see how individual men-tal health and community mental health are intricately connected. Marsha dove deep into statistics and historical research to seek the context that would explain how investments in neighborhood revitalization amount to invest-ments in community health. Each piece also prompts us to consider who our institutions value despite COVID's threat. Dominick and Marsha's reflections show us that in housing the valued are whites, not poor people of color, while Anthony cautions us against getting comfortable in a society where the val-ued get health care and the devalued die without it. Now, more than ever before, the courage they have to write what they see from where they stand is the sociological gift I want my students to have.

Whether virtual or in person, the classroom is where I most easily and frequently tell my own story. During the pandemic it became part of my heal-ing. In early March 2020 as COVID-19's threat became obvious in Europe, my partner and I both started showing symptoms. Days later a doctor virtually confirmed our fear: we'd contracted COVID-19. What followed were harried weeks that went by in a haze of fevers, medicine, care packages from friends and family, coughing, brain fog, and seemingly endless fear and anxiety. During this first bout with COVID—I would test positive again twice—I logged in to a virtual classroom, determined to be resilient despite my own health and the issues my students were struggling with. Some students had their lives upended after being deemed essential workers, while their paychecks and job treatment remained the same. Others had lost loved ones or were suddenly catapulted into caretaker roles. Most were unable to complete their work and reported feeling despair and isolation. At first, I pushed through, trying to keep some semblance of normalcy for myself and my students. I soon retreated from that approach. Though I had always thought of myself as a considerate professor, what my students needed now was an unprecedented level of support. I struggled with meeting that need but persevered and even took on an additional role on campus training faculty to teach online.

I altered classes making space for us to release when we wanted and escape when we needed to. I poured myself into figuring out how to keep students engaged online and how to establish strong instructor presence. I tweaked my syllabus and made myself more available. I was functioning at a high level at a time when my own depression and anxiety were severe. I sought help and a therapist confirmed what I already knew. "You know you're depressed, right?" But I had too much to be grateful for to be depressed, I countered within myself. I was a tenure-track assistant sociology professor, working in a department full of people I respected, in a city I called home, living near many of my loved ones. I was a first-generation college graduate and seemingly living proof that the American dream was still achievable.

During the pandemic, I did not experience financial disruptions even though my partner was forced to leave a job that directly threatened his health. We both had health insurance and were able to see doctors and get prescriptions without concerns about cost or access. My mother became an essential health care worker overnight with little fanfare or change to her income. A member of a vulnerable group herself, she worked long masked hours at a nursing home under frequently changing rules but thankfully, did not fall prey to COVID. Though I knew many who lost loved ones, I was spared that fate. That privileged vantage point led to more guilt and more work commitments to overcompensate for it. I couldn't see the forest for the trees. I couldn't see where I stood.

The autoethnographies in this book serve as pellucid evidence that a multiplicity of standpoints is how we evaluate our existing institutions. It is how we make sure that answers to the question, "How does our society handle_____?" are not shaped by ideologies that rank us by order of importance for access and sow inequality as the consequence. If this pandemic is to serve as a portal, then it must be bolstered by a revolution in our values before it is reflected in our ways of seeing and being as a people and as individuals.

Our sight and our range of motion are therefore inextricably linked even while recognizing that obstacles to our awakening are plenty. These hurdles include neoliberal policies and scarcity myths that harm the truly disadvantaged, growing misinformation and propaganda campaigns, attacks on the LGBTQIA and trans individuals, rising racial tensions and the rescinding of women's rights, ramped up militarism and second amendment abuses, and deteriorating material conditions and life expectancies. The list is endless but so are the possibilities for transforming our world.

Seeing our world through the perspectives of people from diverse backgrounds and embracing the truth-telling in stories like the ones featured in this book are how we start on the path toward a more equitable society. In *Teaching to Transgress*, bell hooks writes that the misinformation we encounter and our addiction to lying about our personal lives means "our capacity to face reality is severely diminished as is our will to intervene and change unjust circumstances."[6] This is why I return to the classroom as the place I feel the most like an activist, where I see myself most clearly, the place that grounds me in my standpoint and encourages me to share my truth and create space for my students to do the same. If the next steps are about how we remedy these evils, then the time I spend with my students, challenging their worldviews and mine, developing our critical lens, introducing us to a range of thinkers and ideas, and cultivating our sociological imagination is one origin point for change. That we engage in these acts of intellectual resistance in the classroom as a community is another.

In the epigraph to her chapter on communion in *All About Love*, bell hooks includes the following quote by author Parker Palmer.

> Community cannot take root in a divided life. Long before community assumes external shape and form, it must be present as a seed in the undivided self: only as we are in communion with ourselves can we find community with others.[7]

Our day-to-day lives seem rife with evidence suggesting that a world that meets our needs with compassion and even love is unattainable. Yet such an ethic already exists, and the stories featured in this book prove that. The seeds of a new normal are present when Dominick writes about the community of his neighbors who "look out for each other when in need, whether it's making a grocery store run for a neighbor, fixing a neighbor a plate of food when they need it, or donating clothes to a neighbor's child." It's what led Billie-Rae Johnson to move back home to take care of a mother suffering from mental illness and COVID-19 and Anthony Salazar Vazquez's family to fly across the country to help an uncle start a new life after deportation. It is what leaves Areeba finding the existing rays of hope that signal the start of new approaches to addressing growing mental health concerns. *Until We're Seen* is an essential text to help us reimagine a new world precisely for the ways of seeing it illuminates.

In the fight for a world that reflects my values and beliefs, a sociological imagination is my weapon of choice. It implores me to probe my standpoint and ask hard questions about what I see and don't see from where I stand. When asked if we are "brave enough to imagine beyond the boundaries of 'the real' and then do the hard work of sculpting reality from our dreams,"[8] I hope the record shows our collective response to be a resounding and unambiguous yes. After all, we have the power to shape what our society can be. "Best to try to shape it into something good."[9]

PART IV

Community Organizing,
Mutual Aid, and Struggle

CHAPTER 16

(Need)les and Many Threads: Sewing Community from Pandemic Puerto Rico and Beyond

Daniel J. Vázquez Sanabria

It was Wednesday, March 11, 2020, when CUNY moved classes online and the uncertainties of the pandemic took over.[1] The retail job I worked in the Kings Plaza mall joined the shutdowns a week later. Suddenly, as a college junior with an almost-maxed-out credit card and growing fears (or panic?) of contracting the virus, I became unemployed. I joined a major economic crisis and those I relied on for help were struggling too.

My sister called over video quite frequently during the early months of the pandemic. She made sure I had everything I needed. During these calls we talked about everything from Zoom classes to the stories of narrow-minded customers visiting her workplace unconcerned about the growing global alerts. It became clear later that these calls also served as a space for us to connect and support each other. These moments painted a detailed picture of the kinds of vivencias this tension-filled time was shaping.

This story is about my sister, who continually builds spaces of care in moments of scarcity. This story is also about a colony, Puerto Rico, and the complications the United States presents for islanders struggling to survive. When a pandemic forces us into precarious conditions and, for those already living precariously, pushes us deeper into desperation, it is often hard to stay oriented, continue producing, and care for ourselves. What happens when resistance takes the form of community building and networks of care? How does our interdependence in the midst of a worldwide pandemic inform the systems we create? For my sister, these questions shape her entire praxis. Puerto Rican women were crucial to the forms of mutual aid that helped people across the diaspora survive. Faced with heightened vulnerabilities, my sister sewed the threads of a network of care that was otherwise invisible to the world yet helped many people survive. This piece maps the story of diverse community networks that supported Puerto Ricans during a worldwide pandemic, and through which we developed mutual aid networks across cultures from the peripheries of empire.

(Her)story: Retelling, Restitching

We couldn't wear masks; we couldn't wear gloves . . .

Living in Puerto Rico and working in customer service at one of the busiest airports in the archipelago—which my sister was doing before the pandemic hit—was not equivalent to staying indoors and emailing professors, which is what I was doing in New York once CUNY transitioned to online learning. During the late weeks of February of 2020, my sister's company, like many others, prohibited the use of Personal Protective Equipment (PPE) in the workplace.[2] Their reasoning against making use of spread-prevention tools was based on their belief that it would create "alterations" to the company's brand and upset customers. "The customer is always right" meant employees would have to risk contracting a deadly virus for the sake of preserving normalcy for clientele. Profit definitely preceded science.

Eventually . . . they said:
"Okay, yes. Now you can wear masks."

While my sister's tasks vary, the core of her work is to interact with hundreds of strangers. When the World Health Organization declared COVID-19 a worldwide pandemic, it became obvious to her and her coworkers that PPE was necessary for ensuring their collective safety.[3] However, the extreme shortage of protective gear during the height of the pandemic made access close to impossible.[4] In Puerto Rico this shortage was heightened because purchasing PPE was blocked by the Jones Act, a twentieth-century law prohibiting the Puerto Rican government from buying anything that does not come from US ports of exchange.

Even in times of crisis, Puerto Ricans in the archipelago are left at the mercy of Congress to bypass or temporarily amend imposed policies. Similar to when Hurricane María hit, Puerto Rico once again experienced a delay in obtaining necessary products because, while "states can break [the rules]" set forth by the Jones Act, the same does not apply to a *colony*.[5] In pandemic times, this meant that the island's sole nonvoting representative in Congress would have to beg FEMA for an exception that would allow Puerto Rico to buy from non-US sellers. Although permissions were granted, delays produced excruciating anxieties among many people, especially front-line workers like my sister.

By the time that happened masks were pretty scarce.
I was able to buy a pack at the Duty Free in the airport for . . . thirty dollars.

It was not until April that my sister's company belatedly allowed employees to wear face masks and other forms of PPE. However, the already-acute PPE shortage made following the company's recommendations a challenge. The airport's duty-free shop was one of the only places with masks in stock at the time, but whose safety was being prioritized when inflated prices made the masks prohibitively expensive? One expensive pack had to serve my sister for everything from supermarket trips to helping out our aunt and grandmother joining the lockdown on the other end of the island. It was then that my sister decided she needed to begin sewing her own masks.

From Hand Sewing to Mass Production

We're going to have to make our own masks . . . so I began experimenting. I was doing research online, and my science background from college went into full gear at that point.

Her first face masks followed a very basic outline and would take almost an entire day to produce. They required only two sheets of cotton fabric and a pellon sheet, a fabric later recommended by health agencies, in the middle to be carefully sewn together. However, the masks were simply meant to keep her and her partner safe from clients who, many times, lacked proper hygienic practices or refused to wear their own PPE during their travels. Realizing a greater supply was needed, she found leftover fabrics, from projects she planned on completing for our baby niece, and began a mass production project.

The people at work were asking: "Can you make me a mask?"
I said, "I don't have that much fabric left over but, yeah, I'll muster something up."

Almost immediately, the fashionable face masks made with "Baby Yoda" and "Star Wars" prints became the buzz of the workplace. Coworkers would approach her about the quirky face masks she wore, and before she knew it, she had more orders than she could produce by hand. It was then that her partner decided to buy her a sewing machine to replace the old and damaged one she owned. Now, my sister was able to produce dozens of face masks within hours. This also allowed her to produce effective Olson face masks, one of the many hospital-approved face masks.[6] What started as a means to protect herself at work quickly became a community project. Through word of mouth and online reactions to her creations, the project also expanded beyond Puerto Rico in an international anticolonial network.

Sewing Diasporic Networks

In no time, this community effort surpassed national boundaries and stitched its own ties through *la diáspora*. One week, while showing me her orders she said: "*I have todas estas órdenes del primo mío allá en New York. He works for the MTA y varias de sus amistades han muerto. Está grave la cosa.*"

She was sending face masks to her cousin, an MTA worker, just a neighborhood away from me. Her reach was quite expansive. It turns out that word of mouth and a little *chisme* here and there gets economies moving too. After seeing him with the masks she had created, her cousin's coworkers, also MTA employees, began placing their own orders. The biggest order she completed for them included more than thirty masks, and the demand grew.

While her prices remained low (under ten dollars per mask), people often tipped her generously. The only reason I know this part of the story is because

I was her cashier. People who ordered face masks from outside Puerto Rico would send me the payments via Venmo and I would later send it to her through ATH Móvil, the Puerto Rican alternative. *"Parece que estamos funneling money,"* I would tell her. These additional payments not only helped her but assisted me as well. *"Quédate con eso pa' que te compres something to eat,"* was probably the message I received the most from my sister during the month of May in 2020. She found a way to both make up for her lost wages and ensure that I had a full pantry.

Sewing the World Wide Web

Mutual care allowed for the emergence of online networks through websites like Etsy and Facebook, which facilitated the acquisition of materials that were scarce or of low quality on the island. Here, information was shared and relayed transnationally between women. Questions about various matters from the availability of materials in any given store to best practices found answers in these online communities. It was here where HEPA filters (found in AC units) proved to serve as efficient makeshift filters against germs and other air particles.

While online spaces were important, some materialized into much more. A childhood friend of my sister's who reconnected with her during this time after seeing her posts online helped find and send materials all the way from North Dakota. Her friend was able to pick up online orders she would place at stores like Joann Fabrics, and ship them to Puerto Rico in what was sometimes a less-expensive and more time-efficient procurement process.

The advantages of this transnational network that stretched all the way to North Dakota allowed other women in Puerto Rico to benefit as well. Once the materials arrived, usually including multiple or overestimated orders, my sister would take what she needed and either exchange the surplus with some friends or sell it to others, who also conducted their own sewing projects. Now, when materials were either unavailable or scarce, my sister could easily leverage her resources and networks to ensure that others had materials and she was not the only one in her area producing masks, which allowed her to control her workload.

Shared Colonial Experiences

There were people in the reservations who were letting us know:
"we need so many masks at this place, we need so many masks at this other place."

This community care project expanded to reach highly vulnerable communities too! After seeing the news that the Navajo Nation was among the communities most deeply affected by the pandemic, my sister, mom, and I devised a plan to send a few care packages with face masks made by us.[7] While video chatting and watching my sister work in her "little workshop," as she often jokingly called it, I learned how to use my own sewing machine. She taught me how to thread the machine, adjust the settings, and select my stitches as I built face masks in a corner of my tiny Brooklyn bedroom. These moments allowed me to appreciate solidarity in a way that also nurtured my relationship with my sister.

We were not only bonding as our machines threaded fabrics together, but we were also stitching on a long history of Puerto Rican transnational support for Indigenous peoples. Like colonies, reservations face bureaucratic (and colonial) challenges when it comes to sustaining and expanding their economies. Despite a series of treaties signed throughout history, the US government failed to efficiently direct resources to tribal governments in the height of the pandemic which forced native nations to take drastic measures to reduce exposure levels.[8] During this time, outside assistance arrived before the US government, including when South Korea sent ten thousand face masks and other pieces of PPE to the Navajo Nation.[9] This, along with smaller scale responses, are what upheld many Indigenous communities, demonstrating the power of long-standing solidarity networks created by shared colonial experiences.

In total, we each managed to send two care packages to the Navajo Nation in Arizona. While my newly found mask-making skills did not allow me to produce large numbers of masks, my packages were sent with thirty reusable masks in one, and a few boxes of disposables in the other. My mother was able to produce almost forty masks and my sister, who was the most skilled of us, sent two packages with forty reusable masks each along with a few boxes of disposable ones. The impact of our efforts was later reinforced with the CBS production of the documentary series of "Coronavirus in Navajo Nation"

(2020) which featured Dr. Michelle Tom, who facilitated our donations and was introduced to us by some of the directors of the Urban Indigenous Collective, a New York City organization.[10] Through all of this, my sister and I reflected on our experiences as Puerto Ricans, building community and caring for one another beyond the archipelago.

Detangling Knots

Most of the island was not ready . . .

Efficient governmental response is foreign to us Puerto Ricans. Community efforts that arise as a result of this negligence are lifesaving. Responding to crises from the periphery of empire is a collective effort. Shared colonial experiences make our survival a shared one as well. In actuality the colonial period never ended. Despite a change in management when the United States took over after Spain in 1898, Puerto Rico remains a colony today. Yet, the underestimation of Puerto Rico's ongoing colonial reality erases violent experiences like the ones documented here. Few stories from the pandemic have emerged from the Caribbean, leaving out places like Puerto Rico or the Virgin Islands from the general picture. Whether it is building a hospital for Vieques—a project continuously delayed since 2017—or ending food insecurity on the archipelago, the United States has failed in the most basic of tasks: keeping its citizens alive and well.[11]

Indeed, the pandemic offered a clear reminder that citizenship is not enough to keep us alive. In 2020 and 2021, when countries closed their borders to foreign travelers, the façade of legal citizenship did not ensure safety for Puerto Ricans. The island's main international airport remained open, and tourists flooded in; for the first time in history, a flight from Orlando to San Juan became the busiest in the world.[12] And although the COVID-19 response on the island has often been regarded as "one of the strictest measures imposed in the US," this too was displeasing to Puerto Ricans. To leave "Puerto Rico open for travelers," as government banners read throughout 2020, allowed US travelers to make the island their own little getaway in the middle of a crisis, while the health of Puerto Ricans remained a secondary concern after corporate profits.

How We Survive . . .

Surviving in a colony is an endless and arduous task. When the state fails, communities of color have already expected it to. While crises and uncertainty have flooded our lives, keeping up the threads that hold, pull, and stitch us together is not merely how we survive. It is how we imagine and build futures that embrace our mutual care, and, most importantly, systems that allow us to stop and rest alongside those with whom we may no longer share physical space but with whom we nonetheless maintain diasporic relationships. A pandemic might have harmed us, but communities of color learned long ago to forge a politics of collective survival.

While stories like this demonstrate the crucial role of interdependence during a global pandemic, Puerto Rican experiences shed light on the obstacles that keep us from achieving and preserving such a life praxis of care. In doing so, stories of Puerto Rican women collectively sewing PPE and creating economies of care allow us to imagine a world where life prevails over profit. Although a way out of this pandemic will not lead us to the comfort of a normative past, overcoming it through frameworks of interdependence and relating beyond colonial borders may serve as a catalyst for new collective challenges to colonialism as an ongoing system and the gendered, racialized, and ableist ways of living it encourages.[13] Sewing a future together in the present is our way out of it all, but only if we are open to embracing each other (despite the forces that claim our differences are too many) to recognize the threads that already tie our masked breaths together.

CHAPTER 17

Everybody's Gotta Eat
(It's Something My Dad Says)

Genesis Orea

I had become familiar with worrying about my father's life.

My parents and I were having dinner and the look on my father's face, a look I had never seen before, was alarming to say the least. He kept clearing his throat, and his face was closer to red than his tan complexion. He looked uncomfortable and when he would catch me glancing at him worriedly, he would just smile awkwardly in an attempt to ward off my concerned look. We were all terrified: this was the second week of March 2020 and the rapid growth of COVID-19 infections in New York City was startling. The city had no idea what was coming, and neither did I. I told my dad, with all the strength I could muster, that I was taking him to urgent care to get him tested for COVID. We were all going, I said. My father, a macho Mexican man, tried to wave off my concern, stating that all he had was a fever and not to worry. But of course, I was worried for him: I had never seen him ill like this, and it had only been two months since his prostate cancer surgery. His immune system was compromised, and decades of chain smoking and his age definitely didn't ease my worries. I knew the look on my mom's face too well; she knew something was terribly wrong. How is it that moms always know everything? I couldn't help but think the worst, because truly, what made my family any different from others who had died from COVID?

My parents were born and raised in Mexico and immigrated to the United States in the 1980s. My father came to Brooklyn and my mother to Los Angeles. As the language broker for my parents, I filled out the paperwork at the health clinic and went into the exam room with my father, for he was the one I was worried about the most. I made sure to train my mom what to say to the doctor when she would see them, because I was also very worried about her, even if she had no symptoms. I tried not to look at my dad who was seated on the examination chair, so he wouldn't see how incredibly anxious I was. Finally, the doctor came in, and my dad looked at me, that was my cue. I told the doctor everything I knew with my dad behind me nodding to confirm what I was saying. The doctor said it probably wasn't COVID but he would test him if my dad wanted; it was almost time for the clinic to close for the day, and they only had two tests left. I looked at my dad's doubtful face but at that point I didn't care about his fear of being prodded by the doctor—I needed him to be okay. I said yes, he'll take the test. When the doctor left to retrieve the test, I comforted my dad telling him that the test is just to make sure, and it's important we know to protect us in his family and those he works with. Thankfully, he saw reason in what I said and agreed.

I told my dad the cotton swab is going up his nose and not to move or else the test wouldn't work. He complied and suffered through the uncomfortable feeling of what he would later describe as a Q-tip going so far into his nose, he swears it touched his brain. The doctor told us it would be a week until the results came and it would be best for my dad not to go to work, just in case. That was the biggest worry for my dad: he has no benefits or sick leave and never misses work. When he had prostate cancer surgery, it took a lot of convincing from my family and his doctor to get him to stay home, seeing as a whole cancerous organ was removed from his body. This time, he finally relented and called in sick for the next day after taking the COVID test. Thankfully, his boss was okay with it and didn't threaten to fire him. My parents are among the millions of low-wage immigrant workers in this nation for whom there is no safety net.

Nine days after my father had his nose swabbed, his phone rang, and I knew before he even answered that he was COVID positive. He quarantined in my sister's childhood bedroom where the most consistent company he would have would be his never-breaking fever and occasionally our dog. I was kept company by never-ending worry and budding mental health issues. Every night I would press my ear against my bedroom wall, the wall my sister's room shares with my own, and pray I wouldn't hear my dad cough. I was scared that if he started coughing, it would mean the beginning of the end, since there's only so much magic Mexican home remedies can work for respiratory distress. Once I heard nothing but the creaks of his bed, I would disinfect our house and my mother's belongings, since she was the one going out to work. She was at risk, and I couldn't risk losing her. As I would sit at my desk and try—and believe me I tried—to gather up research for my senior thesis, I would dissolve into tears. I couldn't fathom what was happening, I was scared I wouldn't graduate without my dad and at that point in my academic career, I wasn't even sure I would graduate at all. As the good Catholic daughter my mother raised me to be, I prayed. I prayed my father would get better, that my mother wouldn't fall ill, that my sister would survive, that I would graduate, and that my community would remain resilient. Worrying about my schoolwork was second nature to me as a senior, but at that point, worrying about school seemed so small in light of the pandemic. I didn't know if the people I loved would make it, so it was quite hard to focus on something like weekly readings. Even when I was able to take two weeks off work with the help of my job's COVID-care policy, I knew that getting paid time off to care for my father was a luxury that most of my community didn't have. They had to brave the front of this pandemic.

While I was taking care of my father, I still had to worry and work with my community. I was working with Mixteca, a Mexican organization based in Sunset Park, Brooklyn, which was founded in 2000 to equip, empower, and enrich the Latinx community in Brooklyn and beyond. Sunset Park's population is about 35.6% Latinx folks.[1] Prior to COVID, Mixteca ran know-your-rights workshops, hosted the Mexican consulate for things like passport renewal, and ran health workshops, financial literacy classes, English classes, and art classes. I've known about Mixteca since I was a child; it has been a big part of my community and the pandemic highlighted not only its importance but its necessity. When COVID hit, Mixteca quickly collected funds from donations and distributed one hundred and fifty $250 Visa gift cards to community members on the basis of need. The truth was the waiting list was over a thousand people, and they were all in need. As I dialed my twelfth person to offer a gift card, I considered myself pretty seasoned as a caller, especially since I had a script. But I was not prepared. I wasn't prepared for people to unload their pain, cry over the phone, or thank god for my call. I especially wasn't prepared for Oscar's story.

Oscar said a fervent "yes" when I asked if he wanted the money. Oscar had been out of work for weeks; he was undocumented so he couldn't receive unemployment or state emergency relief funds. He started collecting bottles on the streets to make money, despite knowing how dangerous it was touching other people's trash during the pandemic. I called him right when he was walking to get his first full meal in days. He told me he was starving. He had been in this country for over twenty years, and this would be the first time he wasn't able to send money to his mother back in Mexico. He told me in tears how his mother would cry for him, hearing the anguish and depression in her son's voice relaying to her that he has no job and no idea when he'd have money to send. Oscar was forced to take in a roommate in the room he was renting in an apartment where the landlord kept demanding his rent. In tears he told me how his back hurt because he would just lie in bed all day, not used to not working, and that he wanted to work. I muted my phone so he wouldn't hear my shuddering breaths as I tried to hold in my own tears, because what Oscar really needed at that point was someone to hear him, just to listen to him.

Gone was the script and my practiced responses. Oscar needed empathy and I tried my best to convey that through the phone call. As Oscar made it into the Burger King to get food, he was too shaken up with either emotion or exhaustion to even try to speak English to the cashier so he asked me if I could tell the cashier his order. I, of course, said yes. Even as Oscar ate his meal, he talked to me, crying over the phone. His pain was sometimes physical and sometimes mental. There wasn't a silver lining to hold on to; he had few to no options available to him. He asked how the Visa card worked, which was a common question among the recipients seeing as many undocumented immigrants tend to deal with cash for fear of any interaction with anything remotely governmental. I assured him he could use it anywhere that accepted debit cards and he would be able to finally buy food with it.

It's one thing to read the stories of people who are less fortunate. But the truth is this is more than just a sad story. It's a reality that millions still have to face in this nation where there is no true empathetic regard for basic human rights. I listened to dozens of community members who were just being told day in and day out to stay home because Sunset Park was a COVID red zone, and they were the contaminants. These people struggled and suffered for the lack of attention they were deemed unfit to receive. This lack of attention plays out in lack of aid and the fact that people in power didn't even think about the lack of systemic infrastructure set in place for something as monumental as a pandemic and what that would mean for immigrants. Despite being the backbone of this city, despite being the cooks, the service workers, the domestic workers, the nannies, the delivery people, the mechanics, the grocers, and the cashiers, immigrants were being treated as if they were disposable. My community was expected to work yet they remained almost invisible unless it was glowing red on a COVID contaminant map. Blame was shifted to our uncleanliness and the refusal to stay home. The fact is there were no safety nets set in place for immigrants even before the pandemic. The pandemic just highlighted an already-broken and racist system that has always existed and always taken advantage of immigrants.

This was the beginning of the pandemic, and the people weren't worried for those who delivered their food and the people who cleaned their homes. To most New Yorkers, these people were faceless and nameless but in a few weeks' time were given the title of "essential." As if they weren't essential before. My mother, a domestic worker in Borough Park, worked through the entire pandemic. Despite her husband and daughter being sick with COVID, my mother couldn't stay home, because staying home meant she couldn't get paid, and not getting paid during these trying times was simply not an option. As I would watch her get ready for work, I would make her an herbal tea, hoping that with my well wishes and intentions, she wouldn't contract COVID. I can guarantee at least once a week I am left baffled by my mother's resilience and strength and yet as her daughter I know where it came from. Given that my mother has no unemployment benefits since she gets paid in cash as most migrant domestic workers do, she was well accustomed to finding ways to feed her family. This pandemic was not going to stop her, neither was the fact that her husband was bedridden, or her eldest daughter quarantined and away from home. Letting her fears and anxieties stop her from providing for those she loves most was out of the question, as it is for many mothers. My mother, alongside many migrant mothers in my community, had to continue to care for their families in a time of uncertainty by rationing provisions that they could barely afford.

Behind every crying ambulance would be a delivery worker on their bike in a rush to get to their delivery. There are approximately eighty thousand delivery workers in NYC, and they have no safety net, no labor unions, no real care in place. These workers' livelihoods and survival were uncertain, and the odds were stacked against them. At every half-empty grocery store, there would be a cashier with no sick leave. I would hear my community suffer yet no one heard their cries or pleas. Immigrant workers have always worked in the front lines, and the pandemic made their jobs harder with either the same pay or less, despite the deeply dangerous conditions. This country has relied on the work of immigrants and targeted undocumented immigrants for decades dating back to the Bracero program and long before. While millions across the United States were ordered to stay home in 2020, truthfully, that was a luxury. My mother wasn't able to stay home; with my father bedridden and money always needed, she had to work her regular schedule as a house cleaner for multiple families. The title of "front-line worker" was far from honorable. Sometimes it felt like a death sentence, said my sister who worked as an emergency room nurse throughout the pandemic.

There are approximately eleven million undocumented immigrants in the United States, and they are unable to collect unemployment or pandemic relief funds, which yet again leaves them to suffer while being taken advantage of. Although four in five undocumented migrants were working in front-line jobs nationwide, there was little to no safety net in place to help them.[2] New York City food pantries and soup kitchens saw a 71% increase in undocumented immigrant clients during the pandemic. There was always some article popping up in my social media feed with hope or a possible chance that some mayor or governor like Andrew Cuomo, Lori Lightfoot, or Gavin Newsom would consider protecting migrants during these hard times. But this was all talk considering many of these motions needed to be voted on, and undocumented migrants aren't really all that popular nationwide, especially if they want human rights. Round after round of federal aid was announced and undocumented immigrants were at most an afterthought. They may have been on the front lines but they sure were not on the front of policymakers' minds. New York City was the first city in the nation to actually "protect" undocumented immigrants, yet, in typical government program fashion, efforts to help them fell short, as David Dyssegaard Kallick of the Economic Policy Institute stated: "Under New York's program, undocumented immigrants who qualify for Tier 1 benefits will get a flat rate of $15,600. That's less than the average of $34,000 that other New York workers got in unemployment insurance (UI) if they were unemployed for all of the past year."[3] Yet again undocumented workers doing the same amount if not more work than their documented counterparts received less, if they were lucky enough to be eligible. While the New York State legislature was going back and forth about whether to protect undocumented immigrants in state policy, hundreds of thousands of New Yorkers took to the streets in March of 2021. In protests and rallies, occupying bridges and the state capital, they demonstrated the very real number of New Yorkers who were suffering under the state's inadequate economic relief for undocumented workers. Undocumented immigrant activists and protesters conducted hunger strikes to tell state and city political officials that they will not be ignored and that undocumented residents deserve the safety of housing, food, economic relief, and provisions.[4]

At the height of the pandemic, Mixteca started a food dispensary. As I sat registering people to receive food, I saw families bringing other families just so they could have something to eat for the week. Mixteca joined forces with GrowNYC to give away about 180 boxes of fresh produce a week to families in Sunset Park. At the time we didn't have a concrete number of the families that were in need, but as months rolled by, we finally had a full Excel spreadsheet with over one thousand families that had received food from us. We would also eventually have to organize a system to efficiently distribute the boxes and reach a wider net of people. We developed a ticket system that would also eventually become inundated with the amount of people that needed food.

We had not only food in the boxes, but also COVID stats and "know your rights" cards because ICE was out and about on the streets. The citywide stay-at-home mandate made it much easier for ICE to find people and create even more havoc during these already tough times. We also started providing flu shots on the same days the dispensary operated and had various rounds of monetary aid, and each week more and more people would apply for aid and come to the food dispensary. I saw my community get hit hard, but the hits were consistent with our pre-pandemic treatment. They were used to the political jargon, the false promises, the limited available opportunities, and the "first-come, first-serve" systems that were never set in place for people like them. Pre-pandemic, receiving state funds came with a multitude of rules and regulations that in the end valued numbers rather than effectiveness. While this proved to be somewhat manageable yet annoying, it would become a huge problem during the pandemic. For the fact is, there were thousands of people in need and Mixteca was just one organization in one part of Brooklyn that frankly was understaffed and overworked even before the pandemic.

Facing the onslaught of never-ending bad news and lack of adequate state assistance, our community members knew Mixteca was reliable. The organization provided a safe haven, whether it was an ear willing to listen or help with paying the phone bill. The people in the community of Sunset Park were accepting donations of Pampers, food, feminine hygiene products, school supplies, you name it, all in the name of bettering their neighbors' livelihoods. They didn't voice their anger at the lack of resources available to them, for they were scared of possible retribution by a government that clearly did not care for them. One of the things that will always stay with me about my work at the food dispensary was that people would tell me as they received their box that they were only doing this because they had to. Otherwise, they wouldn't be accepting these donations. Not because it was beneath them but because they were ashamed, they still had pride, pride that had helped pave their way into this country. Yet they knew that pride was not going to feed their families.

The deadly disease that is COVID-19 fused with the deadly symptoms of an unchecked and an unequal system that was never set in place with immigrants in mind. Immigrants are consistently left behind in a nation that values their contribution only if is profitable for others. Yet my community prevailed. In the face of death and depression there was a spirit of hopefulness and togetherness. We come from villages that survived legacies of abuse and torment by corrupt governments, so my community and my people know what it is like to get through tough times. But that does not excuse the unjust conditions that often make survival a lottery. The hope that remains in my community is resilient and everlasting. I hold pride and love to see my community, my family, and my friends hold on to something that has been ingrained in us. We understand our strength in numbers and the beauty of togetherness and unity; even through those dark days, we had unwavering support for each other. The fact that our community members knew that we were available and answering phones, at the church on Saturdays distributing food, and following up with them provided some sense of stability and certainty during these trying times. We were able to find hope and faith in the darkest times of this pandemic, where uncertainty was the only certainty. Where there were tears for those we lost, there was also celebration of their lives and those they left behind. This is what I and many others held onto. It sometimes fades and dims, but the spirit of hope and the light of my community remains.

CHAPTER 18

Black Lives Matter, COVID-19, and a Cyclical History

Adia Atherley

I grew up in my grandmother's four-story, red, Victorian-style house in Bedford-Stuyvesant, which she and my grandfather purchased in the 1970s. This is my family's house in the United States, the Atherley house. This is the first place my grandparents rented when they migrated from Trinidad. My grandfather was a stone mason, and my grandmother did home care work. And after about five years, they made enough money to buy the house and then send for my mom and her four siblings, whom they had left in Trinidad while they gained a foothold in the United States. My mom finished growing up in this house; I grew up here too. When I was born, my mom and I lived on the top floor, my uncle on the next floor, and my grandmother and aunts on the bottom with my cousin.

My family was still living there when the pandemic hit in 2020. Half of the people in our household—my mother, my cousin's girlfriend, and I—were able to pivot to remote work and school while my aunt and cousin still had to work outside the house, as they were employed by Con Edison and as a union electrician, respectively. It was terrifying to see them leave the house each day, especially before we had a lot of information about COVID and we saw so many people getting sick and dying across New York City. We set up a sanitation station inside the front door with masks, gloves, hand sanitizer, and bags to put dirty clothes in. What eventually brought all of us back into the streets were the Black Lives Matter (BLM) protests that emerged in the wake of the murder of George Floyd, who was killed by police in Minneapolis on May 25, 2020. In the days and weeks following Floyd's death, millions of protestors—including my mom, my aunts, and me—flooded into cities and towns across the country, in the midst of the raging pandemic, in what would become the largest mass demonstrations in US history.

While the scale of the protests was unprecedented, for me, they were part of a much longer history—of our family's participation in the Black freedom struggle not just here but in Trinidad, of my own experience as a young Black person of Caribbean descent, and of the interlocking vectors of disease and race in the United States that stretched back to the 1918 influenza pandemic, which I decided to write about for my undergraduate senior thesis. Participating in the protests showed me that a moment of great fear and outrage, like others before it, could also become a moment of community when, at least for awhile, new challenges to age-old problems of anti-Black racism and white supremacy seemed possible. They were also a cross-generational affair. As in my own family, many people came to the protests with parents, aunts, uncles, even grandparents. Many elders took part. This wasn't just a young people's movement, though that's how it was often portrayed.

Blackness in New York City doesn't mean just one thing. It's all kinds of Black—longtime city residents as well as migrants from the South, the Caribbean, and West Africa. The city represents the African diaspora in its entirety—the making of a new culture from all those cultures, the making of politics from all those political histories. In conversation with people I met at some of the BLM demonstrations, a lot of them would talk about how their parents advocated 1990s US Black Power ideas or how their parents had migrated and they owed it to them to try to make a change.

My grandmother always told me to make the change that I wanted to see. She had first begun to tell me about her own activism after the killing of Trayvon Martin in 2012, when I was eleven. I remember how shocked I was because he was a kid, not much older than I was. I remember staring at the television as the news story came on and being confused: how could this young person have been shot walking home from the store with a bag of Skittles? Shortly after, my grandmother sat me down and told me all about the racial injustice that she had faced, and the protests she had been involved in, in both the United States and Trinidad.

My grandmother came to the United States from Trinidad in the late 1970s. Early in that decade, she had participated in what was called the "Black Power Revolution" on the island, which had been inspired by the Civil Rights and Black Power movements in the United States and Canada. When I was young, she told me about her role in the protests, in which young people led a series of marches against the first independent, Black-led government in Trinidad, under Prime Minister Eric Williams.[1] During the 1970 protests, my grandmother had been a community organizer, helping rally people to attend the protests. She recalled violent clashes between the protesters and the police, including one instance where she had to run away from gunshots. A bullet whizzed past a friend of hers and they were caught up in a stampede of protesters running for their safety. The movement's demands were in many ways similar to the BLM movement: equal rights, control over and more representation in local government, opposing official and unofficial segregation, and Black economic and political power. Her father, my great-grandfather, was a police captain. He understood the meaning of the movement, but didn't like the dangerous positions that his daughter put herself in to achieve these goals for herself and her community. But she refused to back down.

My aunt went to Medgar Evers College in the 1990s and gravitated to the Black Power spirit there, so our connection to American Black Power was through her. She took a class with Betty Shabazz. The combination of those two experiences—my aunt's activism through Medgar Evers and my grandmother's in Trinidad—showed me that history is a thing that you study and can also shape.

My grandmother died in 2014, so she did not make it to see the summer 2020 uprisings, but when the protests about another Black man dying at the hands of police brutality started up, I was inspired by her memory to participate. The *New York Times* called the Black Lives Matter demonstrations of 2020 "the largest [protest] movement in the country's history."[2] Civis Analytics polls suggested that fifteen to twenty-six million Americans participated in the BLM demonstrations, happening every day at several locations across the country and around the world. I started checking Twitter and Instagram daily to see the long lists of protests scheduled all over the country, and in New York City.

The first protest that I joined happened when my mother, two aunts, and I were sitting on our porch. We heard voices and a lot of noise up the block. The protest was passing right down my street, and we grabbed our shoes and jumped in. In this protest in the heart of Bed-Stuy, a historically Black neighborhood, the demonstrators reflected gentrified Brooklyn: the large majority were, to my surprise, white. Bed-Stuy is in the late stages of gentrification, and it was jarring to see on the streets the shift in demographics in the place where I grew up. Yet I did appreciate the participation from non-Black New Yorkers as it showed that, while the issue was rooted in race and racism, it was not just a fight by and for Black people alone. This protest was comprised of people holding signs and repeating the chant "Hands up, don't shoot!" This one in particular had a shorter route, kept mostly to the inside streets not avenues, and therefore had a different vibe from the other protests I attended.

A few days later, my mother and I were walking to the mailbox near our house and saw people with signs rapidly walking toward Fulton Street, a central commercial street in our neighborhood. We rushed in that direction to find a well-organized protest with podiums and speeches (some protests were planned, more formal, and meant for a specific area and others were more spontaneous and free-flowing). Many Brooklyn demonstrations ended at the Barclays Center, where the Brooklyn Nets play, and that was usually as far as my mom wanted to go. The protests were exciting, but given the fear around the pandemic, the large numbers of people attending and the presence of the cops, they also made us, like so many other protestors, nervous. I preferred going to protests with my mom so we could look out for each other.

At one protest I attended near the Barclays Center, protestors were all wearing masks, and people were handing out hand sanitizer, masks, and other PPE. There were so many people there and it was the first time that I had seen or been a part of a crowd since the pandemic started. I worried about my health and the health of my mom and aunts, whom I brought along with me to the protest. I did not want them to catch COVID or for me to bring COVID back home with me. We all wore N-95 masks and once I found a spot in the group, as we all collectively walked along Atlantic Avenue, it made me feel like a part of a community for one of the first times in my life. Everywhere I looked, I saw people of all ages, sizes, races, and orientations—all with masks on. I was amazed that we were able to come together, safely, at a time when the pandemic was enforcing so much separation. It was a beautiful thing.

This reality was so different than the image of the protests that news outlets were painting. The attention was on COVID, but it turned out there was a lot more risk from the police and their activities. The police presence—and the ways the protests were covered—had a menacing feel; even when violence didn't happen (which it did sometimes), it was right under the surface.

When I arrived home that day and turned on the news, people were talking about how dangerous and irresponsible the demonstrations were and deemed them "super-spreader" events. In fact, personal space was respected at the marches I attended; everyone knew the time that we were demonstrating was a critical one for public health. The protests took place before vaccines were available, and there were vulnerable people who had preexisting conditions participating. Everyone tried to be as socially distanced as possible, while still showing a united front and a sense of togetherness. After marching in the July heat, I remember how tired my legs felt but also how optimistic I felt about the future of our society. When we finally reached the Barclays Center, there were a lot of police there and we started cycling through chants that were used in the protests for other wrongful deaths in the past like "Hands up, don't shoot!" and "No justice, no peace!" The uncertainty of what the police would do was terrifying, and I felt vulnerable. When I looked over to my left, there was a small child, about five years old, holding on to their parent's hand and waving at me. When I looked over to my right, my mother was there with the sign that she made that said, "United we stand, divided we fall." Even two years later, those are the most memorable moments for me.

It turned out that the real threat to protestors was not COVID, but the police. Several NYC protests resulted in "clashes" between the police and pro-testers. One of my best friends at a 2021 protest near the Brooklyn Bridge was accosted, arrested, and unable to be contacted for hours. She went to protest with her boyfriend and said that the number of police was breathtaking. I think the location made the tension significantly worse between police and demonstrators, which led to the clash. At other times, protesters were practi-cally kidnapped, zip-tied and arrested, and put in vans by police.

The intersection of the COVID-19 pandemic and the BLM demonstra-tions raised comparisons between today and over a century ago. According to the COVID Tracking Project and the Boston University Center for Antiracist Research, the Racial Data Tracker, Black Americans died from COVID-19 at 2.4 times the rate of white people in the first phase of the pandemic.[3] Nata-lia Linos published an op-ed in the *Washington Post* at the very beginning of March 2020 about the problem of pandemics and the possible future of COVID-19. Linos stated that "Epidemics emerge along the fissures of our society, reflecting not only the biology of the infectious agent, but patterns of marginalization, exclusion, and discrimination."[4] The most marginalized groups in America suffer most during health crises—not because of a bio-logical difference, but because of previously existing social conditions like poverty, food deserts, and inaccessibility to proper health care—and with COVID, having to work so others could shelter at home.

This was true for Black Americans during the COVID pandemic and the influenza pandemic of 1918. I decided to research this for my senior thesis, to explore a parallel moment where a health crisis and racism intersected. During the 1918 influenza pandemic, Black people were deemed disease carriers and were said to be biologically different from white people. As a result, African Americans received virtually no empathy or assistance from the white community. In 1908, Dr. Bernard Wolff, the president of the board of health in Atlanta, blamed the city's high death rate on the fact that 40% of the population "is composed of negroes, with their notoriously unhygienic and insanitary modes of living, and their established susceptibility to disease, especially of infant classes."[5] Wolff stated that the health department could not be held responsible for the high death rate among Black citizens because they lacked resistance and were unclean, unlike the white citizens of Atlanta.[6] Disregarding the health of Black Atlantans, Wolff only agreed to improve the horrible environments that the Black communities in Atlanta had to live in because it "affects the city's reputation while threatening the health of white persons."[7] The assistance that the Black community got from health officials in Atlanta was because Black people had contact with white people, such as taking in laundry and cleaning homes, and the officials did not want dis-ease to spread among the white population. The *Atlanta Constitution* stated baldly: "To purge the negro of disease is not so much a kindness to the negro himself as it is a matter of sheer self-preservation to the white man."[8]

Black newspapers kept Black communities informed about the pandemic and challenged the racism coming from health officials. For instance, in 1918–1919, the *Chicago Defender* wrote about the cramped, unsanitary conditions that the police were placing prisoners in during the influenza pandemic.[9] The paper brought up the historically heightened tensions between the police and the Black community and noted that police stations were "doing more to breed disease than any other agency supposed to be working for good in the city of Chicago."[10]

I have always thought that a sort of blame has been placed on Black people whenever death in the Black community is concerned—in the con-cept of "Black-on-Black crime," or gun violence more generally, or police brutality, and now around COVID deaths. When a Black person dies in any of these situations, the victim is blamed: "He should have complied with the officer," or "She shouldn't have run or made any swift movements." In George Floyd's case, drug use and theft were used as reasons to try to excuse his brutal and very public murder. In Emmet Till's case, impropriety toward a white woman was offered as the reason for his brutal killing. The white aggressors are never really questioned or made to feel real guilt for their wrong actions. Whether in 1955 or 2020, a Black person's death at the hand of a white person is always being justified by some previous action taken by the Black victim.

The Black Lives Matter protests of 2020 and 2021 may have been the first time that millions of Americans were vocal about police brutality and social injustice, but the unjust killing of Black people by police officers has a long history. As a Black person living in America, I have been acutely aware of this. What was different about George Floyd's murder was that it was caught on camera and went viral at a time when, due to the pandemic lockdown, there were few other distractions. Videos of other Black people's death, such as Sandra Bland and Eric Garner, have gone viral before, but this instance was different: it occurred at the very beginning of the pandemic, during the first few months of lockdown, when most things that were not essential were closed. People couldn't pretend that it wasn't happening or be too preoccupied with anything else because there were very few distractions. George Floyd's death peeled back the loosely-held utopian facade for many Americans, especially non-Black Americans who experience police brutality at a lower rate. It exposed the racial bias that is ingrained in the police system, and it exposed the people that uphold systemic racism. This could be seen in the way that the police reacted to the peaceful protesters at Black Lives Matter demonstrations as opposed to the aggressive, and at times deadly, white supremacist groups, such as those that stormed the US Capitol on January 6, 2021.

At a time when so many people were dying of disease and life felt so precious, seeing someone's life be taken without a second thought and with little repercussion was too much for a lot of people, me included, to just sit by and watch. This phenomenon of police immunity from consequences propelled many Black people to be as active as they were in these demonstrations, hoping that the noise would be heard by the legal system and something would be done about the criminals that murdered a man in broad daylight. And this time, in the context of the massive protests, the officers were actually convicted and some sentenced for their crimes. I remember the day that one of the officers was sentenced and celebrating with my family and feeling optimistic about the future of proper prosecution for cops when they commit police brutality.

Some people called the BLM protests of summer 2020 a young people's revolution, but it was really multigenerational. People of all ages participated because these issues are part of a long history of discrimination and systemic racism in the United States and around the world. People have been advocating for the end of police brutality for years, across generations, as in my family. Although we celebrated when the police officers responsible for the death of George Floyd were held accountable, the bar is so low that just someone being convicted of their heinous crimes was a win. Racism and police brutality and even COVID are made just barely livable until something flares up and causes a large disturbance, and then still not much is done. And honestly, the protests produced little if any systemic change. There has been little political response; not even a police brutality bill. That NYC's November 2021 mayoral election was won by an ex-cop who favors increased police funding shows just how little progress we've actually made and how little the calls to "defund the police" were taken seriously by politicians. All that protest and only some minimal accountability for a few officers. Breonna Taylor's killers weren't even convicted. While the protests felt hopeful and produced a powerful sense of community, Floyd's death and others that have followed helped me see that no matter the location in the world—Trinidad or America—racism is so ingrained it will take a lot more than one case to change it.

CHAPTER 19

Pandemic Deepens Food Inequality in Brooklyn: Live from Bed-Stuy

Khadhazha Welch

Live from Bedford-Stuyvesant

"I don't know, Mommy, I just find it weird that I have to go all the way to Trader Joe's in upscale Brooklyn Heights to find affordable, fresh food just because the grocery store by our house wants to sell us rotten fruits and milk for over eight dollars." It was the only thing I could say on Facetime with my mother as we talked during the peak of the 2020 COVID-19 pandemic in Brooklyn. My eyes wandered over $3 a pound for spoiled grapes and a 30–50% price increase for meat; milk that was once $3 was now $8.25. Not being the only one dismayed by the sudden price increases, it wasn't surprising to hear other patrons in the grocery store express their grief with comments such as "Since when does this cost this much?" and "Come on, you know no one is working right now; don't take advantage of the people." Price inflation paired with the rise of unemployment left many Brooklyn residents to make tough choices. Usually, most people were able to note a sudden price increase in produce or dairy with no more than a raised eyebrow and a disgruntled grunt because they knew that a steady flow of income would keep them afloat and make up for the extra money spent. But now, as people lost work during the pandemic, every dollar often counted toward securing meals for themselves and their loved ones, and many residents were left with three options: seek food security within local food pantries, buy less food, or if all else fails, succumb to hunger.

Is Healthy Food a Privilege or a Right?

As I voiced my concerns to my mother, it was evident why healthy, more affordable food was accessible in affluent communities where the racial and economic makeup was much paler and wealthier than mine. Food inequality—what researchers call food apartheid (the lack of affordable, nutritious food in parts of the city)—has been a long-standing problem in Black communities and one of the prime contributors to disproportionate rates of hunger. The arrival of the pandemic not only revealed but also intensified food inequality in Black communities throughout America. Sadly, my neighborhood of Bedford-Stuyvesant was among the first to be hit.

Disproportionately affecting Black New Yorkers as food pantries closed across the city, including 58% in my area due to the pandemic, the lack of healthy food access would only aid in the demise of my community mentally, physically, and spiritually. While healthy food access has been seen as a norm for most white Americans, in Bed-Stuy it was seen as a signifier of privilege, luxury, and a clear distinction of class. "Across the city, in neighborhoods that have been most devastated by the virus—which also happen to be the neighborhoods where poverty is greatest—hunger is emerging as the primary concern."[1] According to Food Bank NYC, neighborhoods such as Crown Heights and Far Rockaway were among the city's top ten communities where meal gaps were most prominent.[2] Within these communities, food assistance providers were able to minimize the effects of food inequality prior to the pandemic. Unfortunately, however, due to the spike of COVID-19 in the spring and summer months of 2020, the vast majority of food assistance providers in these communities of need were forced to shut down.

In Bedford-Stuyvesant, the economic loss that intensified during the pandemic presented itself in numerous ways. Many people in the community were left searching for answers. One Bed-Stuy resident, Jemal Clarke explained, "I had to leave college due to the pandemic making me resign from my job at Walmart. When I came back home, I was met with the inevitable decision of choosing between buying basic necessities or going without a meal for the week with the little amount of savings I had which prior to the arrival of the pandemic I utilized to pay my college tuition." Jemal was unable to acquire a job that would guarantee him income and, as a student at a private college, he did not qualify for a stimulus check or for CUNY pandemic relief assistance. Like many other Black and Latino New Yorkers, Jemal felt a sense of hopelessness, wondering where their next meal will come from. Jemal was not alone: according to researchers, "Black and Latino New Yorkers were . . . about three times as likely as white New Yorkers to experience food hardship compared with their white counterparts since the pandemic began."[3]

Recognizing the urgency of the growing hunger problem, people in my community sought to help one another, refusing to adopt an individualistic mindset. Calvary AME Church had one of the few soup kitchens that chose to remain open with enhanced safety precautions to limit the risk of contracting COVID-19. Church members—mainly older Black adults and children—immediately expanded their already established soup kitchen initiative. While prior to the pandemic, anyone who needed a hot meal was able to come inside the church, sit down, and have food served to them, Calvary switched to a take-out model to safely follow COVID protocols. Church members, including my own mother and younger siblings, woke up at 6 a.m. every Tuesday and Thursday to cook and pack home-cooked meals in containers for community members.

Prepared with love, these home-cooked meals consisted of mashed potatoes or rice, collard greens, chicken or fish, vegetables, and the neighborhood-praised cornbread. In March 2020, during the height of the pandemic, church members prepared, served, and distributed 816 meals; this continued throughout the following months. To ensure everyone in the community was fed, church members personally delivered food to homeless shelters, women's shelters, senior citizen homes, and elderly individuals who were unable to safely gather meals on their own. "Our church has endeared themselves to the community even more during these difficult times," Denise Higgins, a member of Calvary AME, proclaimed.

Not stopping there, Calvary AME's initiatives spread to promoting and cultivating holistic living with Radical Living, a grassroots organization which aims to bridge the gaps between healthy food, sustainable practices, and access to green spaces through direct on-the-ground work within disenfranchised communities.[4] Putting their words and mission values into action, Radical Living transformed the Calvary church yard into a vibrant garden bearing fruits and vegetables. Fresh produce such as herbs, corn, cabbage, watermelon, lettuce, beans, and even tomatoes grew outside of the gates of the church. Passersby were encouraged to pluck off and carry home what they needed to curate their own meals. This fresh produce was not only given away to local residents, but also utilized in meal preparation by Calvary members for their community food distribution. Every Tuesday between 12:00 and 2:00 p.m. community members were able to take home up to five containers full of home-cooked food for themselves and their loved ones. Seeing an increase in children within the community collecting meals, up to two hundred meals per week were served.

Denise Higgins notes how appreciative and supportive the small neighborhood where Calvary is located has been of their loving initiatives since the pandemic. The women and children of Calvary were recognized as angels of the community with their warm hearts and kindred spirits, allowing them to limit the spread of hunger that was taking the community by storm. Higgins observed: "We've had members of the community join us on both occasions for our pray walks where we pray and sing throughout the community."

Refrigerators That Bring More Than Food

Despite the city's lack of response to the visible signs of need and decline in Black communities in Brooklyn, Bedford-Stuyvesant residents decided to push the envelope once again by establishing community fridges outside around the neighborhood during the pandemic. Local resident Thadeaus Umpster explained: "It's definitely good timing. Getting this fridge had nothing to do with COVID, but it was just in time," he explained. "The lines are getting longer." The community fridges meant that passersby could drop off food donations at any time and others could select from the donated items: canned foods, fresh vegetables, rice, prepackaged dinners, delicacies and fruits. This expansive range of donations included options that would comply with anyone's dietary or religious restrictions.

This initiative swiftly made a difference in minimizing the rapidly increasing rates of food inequality during the pandemic in my predominantly Black community. A fridge was placed at a neighborhood focal point directly in front of Herbert Von King Park on the corner of Lafayette and Marcy, a short walking distance from my home. This park hosts numerous community events such as movie screenings, school supplies drives, and barbecues. This made the park a prime location for people to provide nourishment to their neighbors. One morning on my daily walk, I was pleased to see local residents, from adolescents to adults, utilizing the community fridge to their advantage. As the lines increased at local food banks, churches, and now local community fridges, I wondered exactly how many of my neighbors and people I casually walked by in my community were going without food amid a global pandemic. Some Brooklyn residents even traveled to food banks beyond the borough in hopes of finding food. As the New York Food Bank noted: "48 percent of Queens-based organizations reported serving clients coming from Brooklyn in addition to Queens residents."[5]

Grandma's Hands

The Campaign Against Hunger (TCAH) is based in Bedford-Stuyvesant. This food pantry, along with its community garden, has been a major staple in the community since its arrival in 1998, providing residents with not only healthy food access but also social services, including SNAP registration, health insurance enrollment, tax preparation, and much more. Unlike most food pantries which provide residents with a set bag of goods, TCAH uses a more holistic and "choice-based approach," similar to a grocery store. Residents are able to go into the pantry and select their own items. This approach not only limits waste, but also allows residents to choose food based on their need, culture, or dietary restrictions. Due to social distancing guidelines, the "grocery store approach" was replaced with a curbside distribution with enhanced safety precautions, allowing residents prepackaged bags of food that accommodate their dietary needs. Despite this set-back, they were still able to provide over six million meals to the residents of Brooklyn after the arrival of the pandemic. Due to their efforts to tackle food inequality, their advocacy and mobilization through their website, ads throughout the community and vocal community support, TCAH saw an increase in private donations and unsolicited grants, was featured on CNN and Spectrum News1, and was gifted a temporary twenty-thousand-foot warehouse space in Canarsie, which is a huge increase from their two-thousand-square-foot food pantry. Partnerships were established with the New York City's Administration for Children's Services and the New York City Housing Authority, with elected city officials providing grant funding to support their initiatives during the pandemic.

Yet support from the city and private sectors slowly came to a halt as COVID-19 declined and the city reopened. TCAH's Racquel Grant drew a vivid picture of the challenges TCAH faces along with their successes. She explained: "Food inequality has been entrenched into the communities we serve and has only worsened amidst the arrival of the pandemic. . . . If anything, COVID-19 amplified what was already happening." These concerns are shared by community-based organizations and residents within the community as well.

Despite a large percentage of food pantries in communities with meal gaps shutting down at the height of the pandemic, funding from the city was delayed to community-based organizations which chose to remain open. This delay illustrates the lack of urgency the city has pertaining to the well-being of Black communities. Residents such as Jasmine Joseph are clear: "The city's overall response to the food disparities in our community has been inadequate and insufficient. Nothing of note can be said about the way that the city has proactively tried to assist with the food inequality issue. Community members have been giving assistance with pantries and soup kitchens, but the responsibilities fall heavily on those small program leaders with very little guidance or oversight. One hundred percent of the credit goes to citizens for doing their part with these programs with what little resources they get. My mother runs a program in Flatbush, and she literally had to shut down the program for like two months because the city said they didn't meet health standards but didn't give them any real guidance on how to fix the issues. Basically, they just said this is what's wrong, you guys figure it out, and that we did, but so many families were inconvenienced because we just didn't have help."

Conclusion: Fall 2021

In the months following the height of the pandemic, it felt as if a veil was lifted from the eyes of residents in my community. Prior to the pandemic, food inequality, medical racism, and the lack of care and empathy toward Black New Yorkers was a known fact, but it was often disregarded under the guise of "it is what it is." The pandemic not only intensified preexisting issues, but left many of us with a heightened sense of community, ridding us of individualistic mindsets. The phrase *Turn to your neighbor*, which is shouted at my local church podium every Sunday, took on a deeper meaning during these troubling times. "It is definitely the effort and work of our community members," Bed-Stuy resident Amanda Ruiz explained, "that ensure kids, families, and the elderly are being fed. I've seen an increase in food drives, food community refrigerators, and food-based events that are explicitly being held by community members and organizations."

Seeing young Black children and the women, men, and elderly of my community risk their lives and health amid a pandemic to ensure the well-being and livelihood of other Black residents was another face of the pandemic that I witnessed. Prior to and during the height of the pandemic, Bed-Stuy—similar to many predominantly Black communities in New York—faced incredibly high rates of meal gaps: over six million per year.[6] Now that the storm has finally passed and the city is presumed to be back to "normal" with jobs opening back up, and nearly half of all New Yorkers vaccinated, pandemic financial assistance programs are halting. It leads one to ask, "Are hunger rates finally decreasing and are residents able to survive without relief from community initiatives or government relief?" The short answer is "No."

Despite the narrative that is being pushed by corporations and city officials, many NYC residents are still hungry and left without means to provide their family with their next meals. Brooklyn is a prime example: despite decreasing unemployment rates in 2021, they are still higher than the state average.[7] These rates were reflected in the ever-growing hunger crisis that Brooklyn residents are still facing. Calvary AME church is among the few organizations that acknowledges these rates and refuses to halt their community food drives. As of October 2021, church members were still preparing and distributing over 100 meals weekly to the community. The continuing demand for meals distributed through Calvary AME further refutes the narrative that residents in Brooklyn and other NYC boroughs are "back to normal" and no longer need nor benefit from government food assistance programs. "Things are far from normal. People are still hungry. I mean, you see it day by day," states Denise Higgins from Calvary AME. "Our aim cannot be to return to the pre-pandemic normal, as that would still leave approximately 1.2 million people hungry and food insecure."[8]

Food insecurity in New York in predominantly Black communities endures due to the lack of empathy and unwillingness to implement policies that will drastically benefit the lives of Black residents. The narrative of NYC "being back to normal" is one that doesn't address the reality of Black residents prior to, during, and after the pandemic. The reality was—and continues to be—that many Black New Yorkers live in communities with food apartheid, food inequality, meal gaps, and overpriced, rotten food for sale.

This is a reality that Black residents are actively working to reverse. Despite being exposed and living through it day-to-day, Black New Yorkers still make it their duty to push for change for their communities, prioritizing that their elders, children and neighbors are fed and do not suffer from the cards that were dealt to them. Food insecurity and food inequality shouldn't have been a burden placed on the shoulders of Black residents during the deadliest pandemic the world has seen in the twenty-first century—nor the responsibility of ensuring our neighbors weren't starving to death. From the young to the elderly, Black residents in NYC not only faced the brunt of the pandemic, but also took on many responsibilities of state officials, who, instead of implementing rightful change within our communities, left us to carry the weight.

CHAPTER 20

On Invisibility

Lawrence Johnson

> I know what the world has done to my brother and how
> narrowly he has survived it. And . . . this is the crime
> of which I accuse my country and my countrymen, . . .
> that they have destroyed and are destroying hundreds of
> thousands of lives and do not know it and do not want to
> know it. . . .
>
> This innocent country set you down in a ghetto in
> which, in fact, it intended that you should perish. Let me
> spell out precisely what I mean by that, for the heart of
> the matter is here, and the root of my dispute with my
> country. You were born where you were born and faced
> the future that you faced because you were black and *for
> no other reason*.
>
> —James Baldwin, 1962

As a middle-aged Black man in the United States, I have to repeatedly swallow the bitter pill that my society, the only one I can claim, will never truly see me—a painful reality I confront daily. This is not an exaggeration but a simple fact. Having lived in Chicago, the South, and currently residing in Brooklyn, New York, I have come to understand two more essential truths about this American experiment. Fact #2: I draw strength from the humanity of those who have nurtured me and the battles they have overcome. My sense of self loses all coherence otherwise. As an idea, our invisibility dates back to

W. E .B. Du Bois's concept of the veil, famously depicted in Ellison's *Invisible Man*. It gains additional significance with Baldwin's insight into how invisibility relies on white innocence—a willful ignorance and denial of Black life embedded within the fabric of America. Fact #3: The COVID-19 pandemic lays bare the racially charged disparities in disaster experiences within the United States in a continued denial of our collective reality.

The authors in this section, Daniel Vázquez Sanabria, Genesis Orea, Adia Atherley, and Khadhazha Welch relate the destruction in their own communities during the pandemic. The practices of community organizing, mutual aide, and struggle are assertions of humanity in the face of destruction. This is a specific human characteristic that Baldwin recounted the day his nephew was born: "It looked bad that day, too, yes, we were trembling. We have not stopped trembling," but fear did not give into despair. "If we had not loved each other none of us would have survived." Baldwin and the students represent a demonstration of how love transforms suffering into the material survival of people and communities. Whether it is Harlem, Bedford Stuyvesant (Bed-Stuy), Sunset Park, or Puerto Rico, there are more authentic stories to be told about racialized communities that are usually misrepresented. The infamous 1965 Moynihan Report, authored by the Assistant Secretary of Labor and later US Senator Daniel Patrick Moynihan, represents the social science standard that targeted the Black family as the supposed source of racial inequality.[1] The blame for Black people getting sick, dying, and losing jobs at higher rates than whites was placed on individuals, rather than the way that laws, real estate markets, and customs organized living spaces that constructed vastly differently lived experiences.[2] The stories about the pandemic in this section are a pivot away from the hubris about the American dream that distracts from real life and an invitation for society and academia to really see American communities.

As a professor, I was stunned by the devastating impact of the pandemic on many of our students. Before the pandemic, during my time at Brooklyn College, I witnessed students often handling challenging situations alongside their studies. However, in the spring of 2020, the severity of the situation reached a whole new level, made more apparent through Zoom. One particular student, Ebony, stood out in my Social Theory course. At the beginning of the semester, Ebony was enthusiastic about using sociology to explore how fitness could benefit young students in resisting negative influences in their neighborhoods. But as the pandemic disrupted the lives of students, Ebony was one of the students I had to reach via text and phone calls to try to reengage them in class.

When I finally met Ebony over Zoom, she appeared stoic, but it soon became clear that the situation was alarming. She apologized for her absence and explained that the Department of Education had reduced her hours, putting financial strain on her, as she was also four months pregnant. Her family situation at home was deteriorating, with her mother having left for Long Island due to health concerns, her father working more hours as a taxicab driver to cover bills, and her brother, without his own room in the apartment, making her anxious about her safety.

She bravely shared her struggles, trying not to cry, and I realized how overwhelming her situation was. Just before our meeting she blew a fuse in her bedroom, where she had moved her essentials, adopting a safety strategy of only leaving when alone in the apartment. She depended on her boyfriend for food and support, but his long work hours in Long Island left her feeling isolated. To add to her troubles, she had poor Wi-Fi, forcing her to exceed her cellular data limits needed for work. I was at a loss for words, not knowing what to say. We switched to the telephone due to the bad connection and this provided the moment we both needed to collect ourselves.

An aspect of visibility is that when you see and know, you are compelled to act. Witnessing Ebony's struggles compelled me to take action. I was most concerned about her access to food. Even though she tried to reassure me that she would be fine and worried about my safety, I insisted that I drop off essential items, including some fruit, supermarket prepared foods, masks, and disinfectant wipes. After addressing this immediate need, like with many other students, we were able to develop a plan to survive the semester.[3] This situation made me realize that there was no institutional mechanism in place to adequately support students during the pandemic. The hidden and emotional labor of faculty and staff, which the college was happy to exploit, was the most significant response to the pandemic.

The Politics of Knowledge

Sociologist Eduardo Bonilla-Silva offers an important critique for how politicians, medical experts, and mainstream media use tropes to perpetuate the idea of a colorblind pandemic. He is one of many academics demonstrating the intersection of the COVID-19 pandemic and systemic racism.[4] However, the student autoethnographies are remarkably different than standard academic scholarship because they are not focused on public figures or academic arguments but on actors in their communities and the vital relationships that are needed to endure. Bonilla-Silva identifies food insecurity and how the narrative of "feeding America" is used by large organizations and elected officials to mask the deeper roots of hunger perpetuated by gross racial inequality. Khadhazha also helps us see that hunger was rooted in racial inequality prior to the pandemic. What we see in her account is the firsthand indignity experienced by having to leave her Bed-Stuy neighborhood to find affordable fresh food instead of rotten fruit and overpriced milk. Whereas Bonilla-Silva and other researchers affirm the reality of disposability that the students document, we do not see the community's response: planting gardens, feeding each other, and making their churches sites for community care. Whereas the social sciences have been overly reliant on statistics, we have failed to document a fundamental reality of marginalized communities, that people band together even more during times of crisis.[5] What we see and do not see, and the larger issue of invisibility, is rooted in who we consider as knowledge producers. The knowledge validation process, Patricia Hill Collins asserts, means marginalized groups have to struggle to make room for their experiences in the academic spaces.[6] These autoethnographies challenge the omission of the particular standpoint of students, who are in academia as learners, but also participants invested in and knowledgeable of their communities.

A serious consideration of these autoethnographies helps us see the invisible politics that are necessary to address systemic racism and a hostile society that requires unique forms of group mobilization and resistance.[7] Invisible politics require an evaluative process where communities make sense of the world from their lived experiences, producing knowledge in the face of state abandonment. All of the autoethnographies are explicit; where the state failed, students' communities, lacking in many basic resources, found their greatest resource in each other and trusted organizations like Mixteca and the Campaign Against Hunger. It is the bonds and trust that Adia described among protestors against state violence that proved more sound than media assaults that described their advocacy for social change as irresponsible.

What I am suggesting is that the autoethnographies in this section represent an epistemological breakthrough. If we commit to our students as knowers, and not deficit learners, we begin to produce a different body of knowledge that can challenge broader narratives that are out of step with how communities practice survival. Unlike other accounts, these writings are inviting us to bring together our mind and heart to fully comprehend what is often made invisible. Herein lies the sociological imagination that Donna Granville speaks about in Chapter 15. We have the capacity to gain insight into our own experiences through the lived experiences of others. Daniel invites us to consider his sibling relationship, their love for each other, the necessities brought about by the pandemic, and the creativity and resourcefulness required to care for others. Genesis invites us to her dinner table and her work in a community organization where she gives voice to Oscar, who is collecting cans while being crushed by despair. Adia's invitation moves us through space and time to consider how familial memory, political struggle, and community are intertwined in a defense against structural violence. Khadhazha presents residents who fellowship through food preparation to address a community's physical and spiritual needs to persist. In each autoethnography, the commentary on the pandemic demands an understanding of human lives forced to respond to their situations. Throughout, love is a binding social force and a serious aspect of the described relationships that is not taken seriously in the social sciences.

These microlevel stories are limited experiences, but they reframe a shared social reality. In "(Need)les and Many Threads," Daniel helps us understand that one response to the pandemic in Puerto Rico resulted in networks used to foster solidarity and care. PPE production against the backdrop of colonialism redefines the US as an empire. This is not a matter of semantics (empire versus nation); Daniel's account of the Jones Act demonstrates how access to PPE signifies a different lived experience in the United States versus US territories. Millions of Puerto Ricans on the island and on the mainland actively contend with persistent forms of domination that define global relations. The metaphor of sewing and threading indicates people stepping in where institutions fail, yet the threads extend to the Navajo Nation and the reality that people experience the pandemic based on their relationship to the United States.

Although not a colony in the case of Puerto Rico, the United States' relationship to Mexico is implicated in "Everybody's Gotta Eat." Genesis Orea walks us through an understanding of how vital Mixteca is as a community organization that immigrants from Mexico depend on to survive multiple threats: disease, unemployment, and ICE incarceration and deportation. In the imagination of the Big Apple, immigrants are hyper-visible as laborers that make the city go but are invisible as people. As a society, we are accustomed to cheap labor, but we refuse the humanity of people who toil. Residents of Sunset Park are cast by a production of knowledge in which social science stigmatizes low-income Mexican immigrants through a "culture of poverty."[8] Culture-of-poverty theories and media-produced xenophobia have stripped generations of Mexican immigrant families of personality and equated them with disease and criminality. This is a weight that Genesis wants us to feel as she experiences the vulnerability of her family, work, and school responsibilities. Yet reality gets more complicated if we sit with Oscar's despair and others like him. The pandemic may not be his primary concern, although he cannot escape that reality. Threats from his landlord, economic hardships made exponentially harder by the pandemic, strained relationship with his mother, the frustration of communicating basic needs, and an injured back all invite us to imagine a horrifying reality where any of us have to contemplate where our breaking point exists.

Yet what does it mean when one is robbed of even small assistance through stigma and shame? Genesis challenges us to understand that Mixteca occupies a complicated space in the reality of residents who struggle with accepting support, "Not because it was beneath them, but because they were ashamed. They still had pride, pride that had helped pave their way into this country. Yet, they knew that their pride was not going to feed their families." This is a quandary that requires us to sit with the micro-dynamics of oppression and the corrosive internalization of personal responsibility. When one's self-worth is based on denying support, simple gestures and accessing basic survival needs are far more complex. I pause to think about the weight that is carried in the idea of the "welfare queen" that was used to characterize Black women beginning in the 1980s.[9] I can recall my own childhood and my mother's pride for not being dependent on welfare and then the shame she experienced when unemployment forced her to accept it. Both Daniel and Genesis help us understand state failure during the pandemic but also the micro-complexities and relationships needed to survive.

Knowledge of Place

Adia Atherley and Khadhazha Welch's autoethnographies are based in the neighborhood of Bed-Stuy. Adia is focused on intergenerational commitments of struggle through Black Lives Matter protests and Khadhazha documents the struggle to feed residents throughout the pandemic and beyond. In Bed-Stuy, like my hometown of Chicago, Black residents exhibit a strong sense of place. I recognize it in Khadhazha's description of the church, its relationship to Herbert Von King Park, and the different reoccurring events that help tie community to a specific location. Bed-Stuy has a particular cultural identity, character, and personal attachment for its residents. When Adia describes her family's home, she is not only conveying her grandparents' move from Trinidad to Brooklyn, but also the cultural significance of owning a Brownstone in a neighborhood that transitioned from white to Black in the 1950s, due to redlining, where Black residents had to rescue it from abandonment. Now Black Brooklynites struggle against gentrification that threatens their neighborhoods' character and generations of life forged through struggle.[10] The residents that they quote, the geographic markers, and the situatedness of Bed-Stuy, in relation to other neighborhoods hold significance and knowledge. Although Khadhazha is focused on Bed-Stuy, she also mentions other neighborhoods with significant Black populations—Canarsie, Flatbush, Crown Heights, Far Rockaway (Queens)—all of them distinguished from predominantly white Brooklyn Heights, where one has better access to fresh produce. Bed-Stuy is not just a neighborhood but the pulse of Black Brooklyn, thus making it vital to the city as a whole and also a metaphor for the treatment of Black life.

"Blackness in New York doesn't mean just one thing—it's all kinds of Black, longtime city residents as well as migrants from the South, the Caribbean, and West Africa," Adia explains. "The city represents the African diaspora in its entirety." Black Power was meaningful to her grandmother because anti-Blackness is experienced in Trinidad and other places where people form community in New York. Residents understand that Black power signifies the empowerment to engage one's local circumstance and the broader unity needed to comprehend anti-Blackness as a global reality. Adia brings us back to Baldwin when she states: "I have always thought that a sort of blame has been placed on Black people whenever death in the community is concerned—in the concept of "Black-on-Black crime," or gun violence more generally, or police brutality, and now around COVID deaths." The politics of knowledge helps us see the conflict in logic. If Black people are the cause of our own deaths, then America can be innocent. If America is innocent, then Bed-Stuy has to be invisible. When people represent their neighborhoods, they are representing their full selves that society refuses to see: their fears, struggles, love, and everything that makes up a community.

Student-Centered Is Community-Oriented

The most gratifying interactions I have had with students in all my years of teaching is when they express that they know that I care and that they have been understood on their own terms. That is what I believe these autoethnographies achieve—the ability for them to be seen beyond their specific community and its history and to relate to others in a recognition of shared struggles, although the specific circumstances may be different.

Since 2020, I have been using Baldwin's letter to his nephew as a starting point for students to express themselves by writing a letter to their fifteen-year-old-selves. After several semesters, I have come to expect that students will struggle with this activity not because they do not have a lot to say, but because at some point in their education, too many have been taught that their lives are not worthy of academic consideration. Much like the student autoethnographies, students in my courses realize that an excavation of their experiences helps them reflect on their families and communities, see themselves in the course of history, and excavate/expose different social issues. It's a messy process in the beginning of the semester, but students from all the different neighborhoods throughout New York City begin to see similarities in the letters that their classmates write to their younger selves. At Brooklyn College, where we talk so much about diversity, when students begin to open up and trust each other with experiences they usually withhold, the classroom becomes a place where we see each other.

In one of my most memorable semesters, when students returned to the classroom following remote learning, our letter-writing process resulted in students forming solidarities around their fears, struggles, and aspirations. The connections that they made with each other compelled them to think about their experiences as students. They wanted to know, after participating in the job talks of Caribbean scholars, why Brooklyn College would only hire one of the candidates in a fledgling academic program, despite residing in the largest Caribbean diaspora in the world. They were enraged, and they wanted answers. In our pursuit of answers, we theorized about power from their lived experiences and the texts that we were reading, and predicted how our administrators would respond to a letter that they wrote to the provost voicing their concerns.[11]

On the day of the Provost's visit to our class, students were prepared with questions to make a convincing case that the college hire at least two of the faculty candidates. I was proud that students advocated for their education and did not settle for nonsensical excuses for why Caribbean scholars should not be prioritized at the college. When students really pressed their concerns and demanded straightforward answers, they were enraged when the provost blamed students for not enrolling in the courses enough to justify multiple faculty lines. After class, they demanded an audience from the chair of the Sociology department who also chairs the Faculty Council, the governing faculty body for the college. They appreciated his straightforward answers about how the structure is set up to prevent social change, but they were done talking to administrators. Inspired to write a letter to current and future sociology students, students spent three class periods discussing how society works, their place in it, and what education at the college should be. With little input from me, they styled the message as a love letter in which love was described as a form of self-love, community building, and collective struggle for a better education.

The letter is addressed, "Dear Students of Sociology,"[12]

The letter begins: "You don't know us, but we love you. We love you when you feel that the world lacks the love that you deserve, and we want you to consider the love that your education needs. Let this letter not only be an eye-opener but a heart-opener as we have been where you are, struggling to gain a higher education and receiving that degree." In making a case for solidarity, they argued: "Tackling the issue of an education that underserves us isn't to be taken lightly. We ask that you stand with us, grow with us in solidarity. Use our experience this semester to move us forward in charting our future, which is also your future."

I observed twelve of the thirteen students in the course actively contribute specific experiences in a general statement about their education. Despite different geographies, primary languages, and socioeconomic backgrounds, they concluded that none of them were educated to change the world, but to find a job. While they all desired meaningful work upon graduation, they were adamant that education should be less about individuals and more about collective interests. That semester they connected to each other in ways they had not done before and in a sense formed a community. They considered the potential for a different type of education that brings people together rather than causing them to succumb to fear and pressure, and education that can transform society.

The autoethnographies presented in this section serve as a model for transformative change in universities across the United States. By prioritizing

investments in students, their education can be enriched through exploring
issues and events that deeply impact their lives and communities. This shift
away from an individual-oriented approach toward a more collective one will
foster awareness and understanding among all of us, bridging the gap between
campuses and communities. Empowering students to bring the voices and
perspectives of their communities into the classroom can create a profound
connection between academia and the real world. By sincerely grappling with
what it means to truly see one another and showing genuine care, we can overcome the fear of self-discovery and uncover new possibilities that are both
remarkable and worth striving for. However, achieving these goals depends on
action and not sentimental intentions. Our future requires a significant investment in education, paralleling the love and support survivors of the pandemic
demonstrated for each other. The COVID-19 pandemic has undoubtedly been
the defining event of the early twenty-first century. To genuinely see and learn
from our past neglect, we must invest in students and communities to be prepared for whatever the future holds.

PART V

Gender, Sexuality, and
Inequality in Los Angeles

CHAPTER 21

"Dónde está tu Ita?"

Wendy Casillas

Multiple times a day I remind my eighty-year-old grandpa that almost two years have passed since my abuelita died, to which he always replies, "No one told me this." I remind him that we attended her funeral, and her ashes are displayed in an urn on top of the piano. But my grandpa persists like she is just tending her orange trees in the yard and will walk through the kitchen door any minute. I have to remind him, over and over, that Ita is gone.

This is the reality of my life as a caregiver for my abuelito who has worsening Alzheimer's symptoms and lost both his wife and son during the first year of the pandemic.[1] Neither my grandmother nor Tio Felipe died from COVID-19, yet for my family, these deaths are entangled with the enduring trauma, grief, and injustice that have accompanied the global crisis that began in 2020.

Before COVID-19, I was living my best life. My partner and I had moved into the guest house on my grandparents' property in the northeast San Fernando Valley. My family has resided in the Valley since the 1970s when my Mexican grandparents decided to make it their home. He, a waiter, and she, a nanny, saved to purchase a three-bedroom house in the working-class suburb of Arleta, where most residents were then (and still are today) immigrants from Mexico and Central America. I live in the same house where my grandparents raised my mother and uncles, and where I was brought home from the hospital as a newborn. This has been a safe space throughout my life.

Before the pandemic, living in the Valley meant commuting for two hours on multiple buses to Cal State L.A., where I was a junior and enrolled as a full-time student. Along with taking five classes each semester, I worked part-time jobs at a movie theater and waffle house to pay my bills. Although I was always busy and exhausted, I was determined to get the most out of my education. I would be the first in my family to earn a college degree.

By April of 2020, Angelenos stopped going to the movies and eating out, and I was unemployed. My grandmother, who suffered from debilitating diabetes and other illnesses worsened by a lifetime of poor access to medical care, asked me to be her caregiver. I would be paid through a state program called In-Home Supportive Services (IHSS), which funds nonmedical care to lower-income elderly or disabled California residents in their place of living, with the goal of keeping them out of nursing homes.[2] This program allows recipients to be "self-directed," meaning they can choose their in-home aides (called "providers"). Ultimately, however, IHSS decides who can be hired and the number of weekly hours of care each recipient is entitled to. I was approved for twenty-five hours a week to care for her. Over 80% of IHSS providers are family members of the low-income people who receive care benefits. In LA County, the majority of recipients are elderly Latinos like my grandparents.[3]

Though I had never imagined myself as a caregiver for the elderly, this opportunity presented a convenient arrangement. I was attending classes online and at home all the time because COVID-19 had shuttered LA. I was grateful to have the opportunity to give back in some way to the woman who had brushed my hair before school when I was young and cooked my favorite dishes like sopes de chicharrones and enchiladas de queso.

Toward the end of her life, my Ita was unable to chew, and I had to blend her meals in order for her to be able to swallow. Living with elderly grandparents and my immunocompromised partner made it too risky to take the bus to bigger supermarkets, as I had before the pandemic. My community had the highest rate of COVID-19 infections and deaths in the San Fernando Valley due to its high number of residents who are "essential workers," and housing overcrowding at twice the city average.[4] Since we live in a food desert, I was forced to walk to the overpriced corner market and purchase what we could afford. There was less money and less food in the house. My grandma lost weight. When I dressed or bathed her, she was embarrassed by her body, and I would remind her, "No te estoy mirando, solo estoy aquí para ayudarte." ("I am not looking, I am just here to help you") Ashamed, she could not see her value to all of us beyond her appearance. My grandma's passing in August 2020 caused my entire family to experience a communal depression. But my grandpa was still living, and his grief accelerated the decline of his cognitive abilities, so my uncle Beto and I had to step in to provide him with round-the-clock care, though IHSS only approved twenty-five hours per week for me.

Two years into the COVID-19 pandemic, the United States is confronting an eldercare crisis. As the baby boomer generation ages, the need for caregivers for the elderly continues to rise sharply.[5] The Urban Institute estimates that "the number of adults ages eighty-five and older, the group most often needing help with basic personal care, will nearly quadruple [by] 2040."[6] The lack of a comprehensive national plan to address the rapidly escalating demand for eldercare has meant that families have had to come up with their own solutions for taking charge of aging relatives.[7] In 2020, over forty-five million Americans (one in six adults) provided *unpaid care* for someone who is age fifty or older.[8] Reflecting society's feminized construction of family care work, including care of elderly relatives, women make up 60% of unpaid caregivers for older adults. The labor done by family caregivers is mostly seen as an obligation that is a part of their family role, leading their work to go unseen and underappreciated.[9] Society does not value care work because it sees it as a private activity that is not associated with the economy. In fact, caregivers often sacrifice their own careers and financial future, reduce their hours at work or quit their jobs, causing new or worsening financial strain.[10]

Nationwide data shows that unpaid caregivers for elderly adults are a racially and economically diverse group, suggesting that this problem cuts across all families.[11] Yet race and social class differences produce unequal experiences among adults who provide family eldercare. White caregivers, and/or caregivers from higher-income households, are less likely to live with the care recipient and more likely to have paid help from nursing home staff or personal home aides. In contrast, caregivers of color, and/or those with an annual household income of less than $50,000, have lower rates of help (*paid or unpaid*) and provide more hours of eldercare that involve intensive activities such as bathing and feeding their relative(s), housework, managing finances and medical care, and transportation. Low-income households, like mine, are more likely to experience high financial strain due to elderly care responsibilities, and caregivers in these families report higher rates of adverse effects of this work on their emotional health.[12]

My abuelito experiences difficulties because of his disabilities, which include Alzheimer's disease and the inability to walk without assistance, meaning that he needs twenty-four-hour supervision and help. Beto and I split the duties of taking care of him, but if you asked my uncle, he would say he does way more than I do, to which I remind him that he and my grandfather live in the same house, whereas I live across the yard. Duties include cooking for and feeding my grandpa, making sure he follows proper hygiene, bathing him and getting him into and out of bed (which Beto does), and keeping him stimulated and emotionally supported. Both my uncle and I are neurodiverse, causing us to experience and exist in the world differently in comparison to neurotypical people. Beto has an undiagnosed learning disability and I have Attention Deficit Disorder (ADD). We often find it hard to do basic tasks that others would find a part of everyday life, such as keeping the house clean and orderly. One of the biggest challenges is managing my grandpa's diabetic diet, which requires meal planning, carb counting and record keeping that is especially challenging for us. There is constant pressure, not just to keep my Ito safe and healthy, but also to avoid negative attention from IHSS. A doctor's visit that uncovers high blood sugar or bed sores could risk our jobs and remove us from my grandpa's care. For all this labor, Beto and I each earn $1,000 per month through the IHSS program.

IHSS caregivers are contracted through a public agency, yet in 2021 we were paid $15 an hour without benefits, well below other public workers. In that same year, for example, LAX airport workers earned a "living wage" of $17 an hour plus benefits or $21.89 without benefits.[13] Not only do Beto and I get paid minimum wage, but we are compensated for less than a quarter of the hours that we actually work. Like other IHSS recipients, my grandpa had to go through an intensive application and assessment process to determine his daily needs. IHSS approved him for only forty hours of care per week, even though he actually needs care every day of the week from 8 a.m. to 10 p.m. (and my uncle sleeps in the bedroom next to his in case of emergencies). The timesheet provided by IHSS only allows providers to log hours between 8 a.m. and 5 p.m., and overtime is strictly controlled. My Ito cannot afford to pay me or my uncle for those additional hours, and the caregiving that we do is made to seem by him and other family members like a favor or our obligation as his relatives, rather than a real job. I do not choose to take care of my grandpa only for the money, but it is challenging to be overworked and underpaid and still expected to work even when I am sick. The income that I earn through IHSS primarily goes toward my rent, a phone bill, credit card bills, and food.

At the end of 2021, my grandpa's social worker visited for an in-home check for the first time during the pandemic. She directed all of her questions to my cognitively impaired grandpa who put a positive spin on everything; in addition to his poor short-term memory, he has a habit of downplaying his pain and struggle. This prevented the social worker from understanding the full scope of his deteriorating health. The in-home check concluded without a recommendation for additional hours of care that my grandfather needed— and that Beto and I were providing without compensation. IHSS's own data show that the state of California is stingy with the care that it funds for low-income disabled or elderly residents. In 2020–2021, IHSS funded an average of 114 hours of care per month for recipients, which amounts to less than four hours per day.[14] These data suggest that most IHSS providers have to choose between volunteering their time or adhering to the hours allotted by the program, leaving the recipient, who is most commonly a relative, without adequate care. The very limited hours that the state assigns to IHSS recipients, and the low wages it pays to caregivers, reflect society's lack of value for low-income elderly people of color.

Since the majority of IHSS providers are relatives of state-approved recipients, this system of employment only works through low-income people's unpaid labor. IHSS treats family caregiving like a side hustle, where providers can work a few hours a day and then go to their "real" job. However, many of us are working around the clock to keep our elders safe and cannot leave the house for another job. Because in-home health care through IHSS is a form of public assistance, the attitude is that recipients (and by proxy their caregivers) should feel grateful for the meager benefits they receive.

The exploitation that IHSS workers experience is typical of the eldercare industry. Research shows that in-home care workers in the United States are more likely to live in a low-income household compared to other workers, and over half must rely on some form of public assistance to support their own families. Across the nation, 87% of all in-home care workers are women, 62% are people of color, and 31% are immigrants. One study in Los Angeles reported that the majority of in-home care workers are women of color over the age of forty-five.[15] These workers, who are taking care of the city's elderly residents, are themselves approaching retirement age without a financial safety net.

The pandemic further exacerbated the problems faced by eldercare workers. Lack of personal protective equipment and insufficient training on infectious diseases caused an increase in fear of exposure for those who worked in-home care, eventually causing staff shortages. Home care workers were

not included in priority categories for COVID-19 testing and vaccination.[16]
The pandemic not only impacted the physical health of in-home care workers, but also strained their mental health, leading many to abandon the field
altogether.[17]

Since becoming a full-time caregiver, I have noticed a drastic change
in both my mental and physical health. I developed chronic back pain and
increased joint and muscle pain. Additionally, my mental health has suffered, in part, because my queer nonbinary identity is constantly negated by
my grandpa through his patriarchal/machista ideologies. He constantly mis-
genders me, using female pronouns, and asks when I am going to marry a
man, even though I am out about my queer sexuality, and he interacts with my
female partner on a daily basis. More recently, as his dementia has worsened,
he has become sexually inappropriate with me. It takes a lot of emotional labor
to provide loving care under these conditions of not being seen or respected.
My depression and anxiety disorder have worsened, and I was recently diagnosed with obsessive compulsive disorder and post-traumatic stress disorder.
According to the advocacy group Justice in Aging, over half of all women who
provide elder care have chronic illnesses of their own. Stress is ranked as the
biggest occupational challenge by one in five elder caregivers and leads to
long-term physical and mental disabilities.[18]

Conditions for health care workers have improved through unionization
and grassroots organizing. Unionized in-home care workers are disproportionately located in the public sector through state-funded programs like
IHSS. In California, SEIU Local 2015 represents over 380,000 workers across
the long-term-care sector, including IHSS and private skilled nursing home
facilities and assisted living facilities. In 2019, the union fought for and won
an executive order by Governor Gavin Newsom to develop and implement a
Master Plan on Aging by 2030, and it is currently campaigning for a twenty-
dollars-per-hour "wage floor" for IHSS workers.[19] SEIU has organized long-
term care workers across the country, with New York's Local 32BJ representing
175,000 members and Massachusetts' Local 1199 with more than 70,000
members. On the other hand, private sector in-home care workers have
been organizing in grassroots organizations through the National Domestic
Workers Alliance (NDWA). The NDWA's "Caring Across Generations" campaign unites elderly and disabled people with caregivers to pressure Congress
to invest in a socially just national system for long-term care. In ten states,
including California, NDWA activists won the passage of a Domestic Worker

Bill of Rights, which establishes overtime, rest breaks, and protection from abuse and harassment. Yet the majority of caregivers in the United States still lack union rights or protections under the law.

As the first university graduate in my family, I had high expectations for what my life would be like after graduation. One year after earning my bachelor's degree. I did not expect to still be in the same position as before I received my degree, I saw higher education as a way to gain more opportunities for myself to grow and expand beyond my own abilities. But so far, I have felt trapped in a cycle of depression and anxiety. The pandemic changed the expectations of life. With so much uncertainty, it has felt impossible to imagine and set goals for my future.

The question always lingers in the back of my head, "Do I have a choice to say no to being a caregiver, or am I unable to say no?" But the truth is that I do in fact have a choice; I make a choice every day to try to deliver the best care to my grandpa. Others might not have a choice because there is no one else who can care for their disabled or elderly family member. Whether or not someone has a choice to be a caregiver, they deserve fair wages and benefits and society's respect.

CHAPTER 22

"In Our Eyes, He Was Everything": Immigrant Fathers, Workplace Regulations, and COVID-19

Maria Cerezo

My fifty-year-old father Refugio Cerezo was a healthy man. He was tall and strong. Before he contracted COVID-19 he worked ten hours a day, six days a week at construction sites across Los Angeles. He knew many building trades, but, like other men in his Mexican family, he specialized in flooring installation. When we were younger, my sisters and I looked forward to Sundays when we accompanied our father to job sites to pick up equipment. He would give us a tour of the house that he and his coworkers were building, proudly showing us the floor materials, colors, and designs for each room. He patiently explained the difficult process of installing different materials—terrazzo, ceramic tile, hardwood—and the artistic vision he had for each project. It was mind-blowing to listen to our father describe his craft and see photos of his finished work. In our eyes, he was everything.

My father caught COVID-19 at work in November 2020. The previous June, when California counted half a million coronavirus cases, Governor Gavin Newsom and LA mayor Eric Garcetti announced that construction was an "essential industry" that would remain open on an emergency basis.[1] While state lock-down rules required most businesses to close their in-person operations in order to slow COVID's spread, construction marched on.[2] Now labeled an "essential worker," my father had to continue working so that our family could pay the bills. Initially after he was infected, my father's condition was stable, and his only symptom was a dry cough. We did our best to follow the doctor's orders to care for him at home. I delivered his meals to the bedroom where he was isolating and woke up frequently during the night to check his oxygen levels and blood pressure. As weeks passed, he got sicker and started to have breathing problems. He lost his appetite and had difficulty swallowing his medication because his throat was inflamed and raw. Talking would set off a coughing spell that left him exhausted and gasping for air. After a month of fighting the virus, my father was intubated in December. Five days later, he tragically passed away.

Doctors at Adventist Health White Memorial explained that all his organs were in perfect condition except for his lungs. Was he a heavy smoker? Did he live with someone who smoked? Through the fog of our grief, my family struggled to understand how a healthy man who had never smoked could have severely damaged lungs. It was only a year later, when I conducted research for this autoethnography, that I understood how my father's work in the construction industry had compromised his lungs and created the conditions for his untimely death.

We have an image of construction workers as young, healthy, and physically fit. In reality, the average construction worker is 42.3 years old, and about 12% or 1.4 million construction workers are sixty or older.[3] At the start of the pandemic, the Center for Construction Research and Training (CCRT) reported that more than half of all construction workers had one or more pre-existing health conditions, such as heart, respiratory diseases, diabetes, high blood pressure, and obesity, that put them at higher risk for severe illness from COVID-19. One in five construction workers had a respiratory disease, such as asthma, emphysema, or chronic bronchitis. The CCRT warned that, "In addition to [pre-existing medical conditions and age vulnerability], job hazards, essential projects, and inadequate health insurance coverage among construction workers could escalate the risk of COVID-19 and have a greater impact on some workers, especially Hispanic and black workers and those employed in high-risk occupations."[4] This warning proved correct, as the construction industry has ranked among the highest proportionate numbers of coronavirus infections, hospitalizations, and deaths among workers by occupation.[5]

My autoethnographic research critically questioned the socioeconomic factors that are responsible for these health vulnerabilities in the first place. Specifically, I wanted to understand why Latino men predominate as laborers in the construction industry, and how this occupation increased their risk of developing preexisting conditions, including respiratory diseases, long before the COVID-19 pandemic. Nationwide, nine out of ten construction workers are male, reflecting the exclusion of women from employment in this male-dominated industry. Latinos are overrepresented in construction work, comprising 30% of this workforce nationally, compared to just 17% of all US workers, and they make up more than half of lower-paid construction laborers, painters, and paperhangers.[6] In LA County, specifically, immigrant men from Latin America comprise almost 60% of the construction labor force.[7] While we may assume that construction work is a stepping stone for young immigrant men who move on to less physically demanding and higher-paying industries as they integrate in US society, in truth, this is an aging workforce; the number of construction workers over age fifty-five doubled between 2000 and 2020.[8] Many immigrant Latinos, like my father and uncles, will work in construction until they retire or die.

In the case of the men in my family, construction was the only employment they could find in the United States because they did not have a Social Security number or speak English. The need to pay back their "coyotes" and send money to family in Mexico pressured my father and uncles to take any job they could get, even if the pay was low and working conditions were unsafe. My father had grown up in Puebla, Mexico, doing physical labor alongside his brothers. Starting at a very young age, he would wake very early in the morning to take care of his family's animals and land. By the time he was nineteen years old, he had worked as a truck driver and picked up odd jobs for neighbors in his hometown. After migrating to Los Angeles, he found work as a chalan (construction helper) for one of his friends, who was employed by a subcontractor. My father, new to construction work, did not question his pay rate or working conditions. The need to send money back home got him to the construction site by 5 a.m., and his experience of physically demanding work from a young age gave him the endurance to move and lift heavy materials, bend over to lay tile, and nail hardwood into place while on his knees.

One of my favorite childhood memories is going to work with my father. Starting when I was seven years old, I accompanied him to his work sites to translate from English to Spanish the site supervisor's instructions to my father. On some occasions, I would sweep, pick-up trash, or bring water to him and his coworkers, but my primary role was to serve as a translator. I now realize that I don't recall ever seeing my father and his Latino coworkers wearing gloves, dust masks, eye protectors, or other safety gear while work-ing. My father and uncles regularly worked with crystalline, concrete, gravel, and heavy machinery without the proper protective equipment. Exposure to these materials is known to cause chronic inflammation and fibrosis in the lungs and other organs, resulting in long-term respiratory diseases. Cheri-yan and Choi's 2020 study, for example, warned of severe health effects for workers who are "exposed at the construction sites," concluding that "their chances of having chronic obstructive pulmonary disease (COPD) are high."[9] The same study found that workers at construction sites are exposed to fresh concrete, dry cutting, and gravel that cause long-term health risks, and at times, workers are not aware of this or are too afraid to speak up.

For my father, getting paid by the job and working from 5 a.m. to 7 p.m. was a respectable way to make a living. Because he was scared of deportation, he never questioned why he had to work without being provided with ade-quate safety gear. After my father passed away, I asked my uncle Jorge, who has worked in the construction industry for twenty years, about his experi-ences with workplace safety protocols. He explained that when his patron (boss) provided him with a dust mask, he would use it, but most often, he was not given basic safety gear nor expected to wear it while working with unsafe materials. His supervisors did not inform him about how working with concrete and crystalline could affect his health. This was information he discovered from talking with his coworkers. Yet, for my father, uncle and many of their immigrant coworkers being able to provide economically for their family outweighed the health risk of their jobs.

This is the case for many immigrant construction workers who are afraid to question the lack of safety protocols at their work site, or who must trade their health for economic survival. A 2011 study of Latinos in the construc-tion industry found that the majority of workers had received little to no training on safety protocols. Comparing the differences in safety training and conditions between unionized and nonunionized construction, researchers found that nonunionized workers hired by subcontractors face the most unsafe workplaces.[10] The study reported that Latino workers "describe cases where they were given inadequate personal protective equipment (PPE), such as dust masks instead of half-face respirators, or no equipment and had to use clothes to prevent breathing in dust." It also specified "economic pressure to work quickly due to piecework pay or production deadlines, lack of appro-priate tools and safety equipment, lack of or inadequate work tools and safety training, economic competition with other workers for scarce jobs, lack of sufficient skills in the chosen construction trade, exploitation and immigration status as contributing to risk and injury."[11]

Gender ideology also normalizes unsafe working conditions in this industry. Specifically, masculinity narratives that value authority, hard work, and prioritizing family interest over self-interest help explain how the workplace culture in the construction industry further magnifies health risks for Latino workers. Saucedo and Morales's study of undocumented Latino workers in residential construction noted that pervasive hypermasculinity narratives motivate workers to accept dangerous and unfair work conditions without complaint. In this workplace culture, men are seen as animals, and because "they are animals, men will perform all sorts of tough, difficult, and dangerous jobs."[12] Their study found that Latino construction workers stoically endure tough work conditions because of the pervasive belief that "a man who complains about the abuse is not strong enough or manly enough to do the job."[13] Furthermore, Saucedo and Morales argue, because traditional Latino values expect "honorable men" to be reliable providers and take risks for their family's security, many Latino brown-collar workers tolerate exploitation and physical harm on the job in exchange for manly status in their family and community.[14]

For all these reasons, the construction industry was a loaded powder keg when the COVID-19 virus emerged. When the City of L.A included construction in its list of "essential industries," close to a million people worked locally in construction, and LA County was expecting to finish thirty-one thousand units by the end of the year.[15] The mayor's office and the County Board of Supervisors saw construction as vital to stimulating the region's stalled economy and alleviating a severe housing shortage that plagued the LA metro area. Demand for construction services grew during the pandemic as local businesses and homeowners saw stay-at-home orders and business closures as an opportunity to get repairs or remodeling done. Residential construction in LA County jumped by 21% in 2021. While employees in other industries were able to work from home, construction workers like my father continued to work on construction sites where new protocols established by the County of Los Angeles Health Department required masking, social distancing, and hand-washing stations.

A 2022 nationwide study found that contractors reported rising costs due to supply-chain interruptions, the need for PPE materials, and additional labor costs due to labor shortages caused by workers getting sick and hiring workers to take on extra shifts and work overtime.[16] The most accessible PPE materials provided by construction employers to workers were latex gloves, hand sanitizers and N95 masks. Health and safety precautions varied widely across company types and sizes, with smaller companies and independent contractors scoring lower on safety measures than large construction firms.[17] Workers often did not question if tools were sanitized and safely stored, which if not done correctly, could increase contamination. A survey of construction workers conducted in summer 2020 found that about half of research participants stated that information given to them regarding COVID-19 did not inform them how to implement safety protocols; training was not informative, and at times, not available in Spanish. Some construction workers also reported that they were not following employer-mandated safety protocols or implementing social distancing, especially during their lunch break.[18] My uncle Jorge told me that at the beginning of the pandemic, few men at his job sites wore masks. Men who sanitized their hands and kept their distance were labeled as paranoid by their coworkers. There was a lot of goofing around and bravado, with many workers claiming that they were not afraid of the virus and only wore a mask because it was required. Regardless of whether it was employers or employees who did not follow COVID-19 safety rules, construction worksites were not safe for workers. In just the first month of the pandemic alone, the City of Los Angeles issued 215 citations and shut down three construction sites for violating public health regulations.

As our family's only provider and an undocumented immigrant who was excluded from federal COVID-19 relief, my father had to continue working in person. But he was fastidious about masking, even when the other men at his job site were not. He regularly used hand sanitizer and sprayed Lysol around his work area to avoid infection. One of his brothers, who also works in construction, taught him to take off his shoes before entering the house and immediately shower and change clothes in order to try to prevent bringing the virus into our home. Getting sick was not a chance my father was going to take.

My father's time in the ICU is one of the hardest experiences that our family had to go through. Because he was in critical condition when he arrived at the Emergency Room, we were not able to say goodbye before he was intubated. The next time we saw him was when his ICU nurse called us on FaceTime so we could see him lying unconscious with tubes and machines around him. My father was a person of strong faith and encouraged us to always rely on our religion during our most difficult times. Every day we prayed together as a family for his fast return and constantly called the hospital to check for any updates on his condition. Nurses would call our home in the middle of the night to tell us that his oxygen levels were rising, and the next night to say that his lungs were not fully working. He passed away five days after being hospitalized.

We were shattered and left with questions about his death that we did not have answers to right away. We were not able to fully grieve at that time because there were so many things that had to get planned and done. My father died during the week of final exams, so I faced much pressure to pass my classes for the semester. After his passing, my sister and I became the breadwinners of the family. I continued taking five classes per semester at Cal State LA, while increasing my work hours at a warehouse to an average of forty per week. In the first two years after my father died, I worked weekends, overtime, and overnight shifts so that I could take classes during the day. My weekly paycheck of $800–$950 helps my older sister provide for our family.

Being able to understand how my father's experience as a construction worker impacted his death from COVID-19 has given me some clarity and closure. I now know that the breakdown of safety measures before and during the pandemic contributed to him being at a higher risk of exposure, like many other front-line workers. As a result of my research, my family now understands that my father worked with toxic material throughout his adult life and that these materials ravaged his lungs. Reading other stories about front-line workers who passed during the pandemic has made me feel less alone. We came to accept that we will still have hard days where we miss our father, but also that we can rely on one another to get back on our feet. We try to remember our father every day and use his values and love to guide us.

CHAPTER 23

"Zoom School" and the Digital Divide in Immigrant Communities During COVID-19

Elizabeth Leon Lopez

"It's Corona time!" sang my four-year-old son, Leonardo (TikTok song at the time) as we prepared for the stay-at-home order caused by the COVID-19 virus. There was panic in the air, and everything felt unstable. Shortly after going into lockdown, my son's school confirmed we would switch over to distance learning for the rest of the year, or as Leonardo calls it "Zoom school," and he would begin his journey as an online Transitional-Kindergarten (TK) student. He was initially excited that he would be doing "school just like mommy." While I am a full-time college student-parent, not a TK'er, I know the struggles of distance learning all too well. I transferred from community college to Cal State LA during the pandemic, so my classes were all online. Since Leo's and my virtual class meeting times conflicted, I had to borrow a laptop from his school for him to use. This is great news, I thought to myself at that time. Schools are providing laptops for children who do not have a computer at home so that they can continue their education. Everything pointed to a smooth transition to schooling from lockdown at home.

"Mommy . . . mommy . . . I need help! My teacher can't hear me!" cried my son with tears rolling down his face as I was putting my two-year-old down for his morning nap. I hurried over to show him how to unmute on Zoom. Then I explained to his teacher that Leonardo was still learning how to use a computer. This was only the beginning of our distance-learning struggles. I realized that I needed to devote more time to monitor him more closely to manage his frustration during school hours. This complicated things for me as I usually would take advantage of my toddler's nap time to get my schoolwork done. But this was no longer an option. While Matthew napped, I had to stay on mom duty so that Leo could attend Zoom school.

I was in charge of the kids because my husband worked full-time as a chassis mechanic, and his job was considered "essential." In addition to caring for our young kids and taking five online college classes, I worked every weekday at a childcare center that stayed open during the lockdown for essential workers who needed a place to send their kids. I worked the opening shift, from 6:30 to 9:30 a.m., which meant I woke Leo and Matthew up around 5 a.m., got them dressed and fed, and drove them to their grandparents' house. After work I would pick up my kids and go straight home to give them an early lunch and set Leo up for online school at 11 a.m.

Nearly four million undergraduates in the United States are parents to children under the age of eighteen, and 68% of these student-parents live in poverty.[1] Even before COVID-19, student-parents faced significant debt, food insecurity, and homelessness. During the pandemic, the psychological and financial pressures on student-parents multiplied, "threatening their ability to keep their families healthy and secure on top of maintaining their studies remotely."[2] I was fortunate that my husband and I did not lose our jobs during the pandemic and that my parents helped with childcare. Yet during the year that Leo's school was closed, I found myself having to choose between my son's education and my own.

As Leo got the gist of using a laptop and attending online school, I gave him more independence with his learning. Nevertheless, there would be days of frustration—not only his, but also his teacher's, who had to manage a class of sixteen four-year-olds in an online environment. Most TK'ers are not computer savvy, and technological access and mastery is especially elusive for primary school students from low-income families who are less likely to have a computer at home.[3] At Leo's school, John Muir K–8 Academy, which is part of the Long Beach Unified School District (LBUSD), over 95% of the one thousand enrolled students are Latino or African American, three-quarters are classified by the state as "socioeconomically disadvantaged" and 10% are houseless.[4] In the first year of the pandemic, school personnel distributed hundreds of Chromebooks and textbooks for students to use at home, set up drive-by stations for families to pick up free meals, and directed them to free COVID testing and vaccinations. The needs of the John Muir Academy community during the pandemic were immense.

The majority of Leo's classmates were Latino children from immigrant households, a group that was disproportionately impacted by digital inequity during COVID.[5] There were five Latina immigrant mothers who attended the TK online class every day to make sure that their child was connected and learning. The teacher only spoke English and the mothers only Spanish, so they couldn't follow the teacher's technology instructions, and the students were too young to know how to manage the computer using the teacher's directions. Despite everyone's best efforts, almost every class meeting devolved into children crying and technological disruptions that impeded student learning.

Latino immigrant families, including my tias (aunts) who are immigrants from Mexico and their primary-school-age children, had to navigate the challenges of online school during the first year of the pandemic from the other side of the digital divide. Due to intersecting inequalities around social class, language access, and technological access and literacy, immigrant mothers struggled immensely to help their young children use Zoom and navigate the school applications for learning materials and homework.

Even before the pandemic, there were an estimated 1.2 million K–12 students across California without internet access at home.[6] In 2019 researchers from USC's Annenberg and Price Schools warned that, "In LA County, roughly one-in-four households with school-aged kids—some 250,000 families—lacks access to both broadband internet and either a laptop or desktop computer." They found that in predominantly African American and Latino areas, like Watts and East LA, over half of households with children did not have full access to the internet.[7] This digital divide was not simply due to lower consumer power among low-income parents, but also because "low-income and 'minority' neighborhoods are often bypassed for infrastructure investments, . . . meaning families in these areas typically have fewer internet providers to choose from—and must often pay higher prices for access."[8] The lack of government and corporate investment in telecommunications infrastructure in low-income communities technologically disadvantages students of color in K-12 and higher education.

When COVID-19 forced the state's public schools to close, the preexisting digital divide became a full-blown public crisis as school districts struggled to acquire and distribute hundreds of thousands of computers and hotspot devices to students. As California's third largest school district, Long Beach Unified (LBUSD) had to rapidly transition to distance learning more than 70,000 students—over 85% of whom are Latino, African American, or Asian Pacific Islander, and 63% low-income. In the neighboring Los Angeles Unified School District, school officials scrambled to get laptops to more than one-third of the districts' 600,000 students, and negotiated with Verizon to offer temporary free internet service to tens of thousands of students whose families could not afford it.[9]

By mid-May of 2020, LBUSD and LAUSD officials triumphantly announced that they had significantly narrowed the digital divide. Devices had been distributed to over 90% of students in need.[10] Schooling could resume from home. Yet for many low-income students and their immigrant parents, like those at my son's school and my extended family, the rupture in educational access and learning persisted long after students took their Chromebook home and connected to the internet.[11]

In my son's school, many of the loaner computers had horrible audio problems or the students did not have high-speed internet at home, which caused the video feed to constantly freeze. With the audio screeching and TK'ers covering their little ears in alarm, the teacher had no option but to kick the student with the faulty computer out of the Zoom meeting. Even though all children in the United States are guaranteed a K–12 public education, the students in my son's class were constantly being ejected from the Zoom classroom and, not surprisingly, struggled to learn in this unstable environment. It became clear that the solution to distance learning for Latino immigrant families was not simply about gaining access to computers and internet service. Rather, the pandemic exposed a continuing deep divide around equitable access to *quality* technology and digital literacy, which scholars define as the knowledge and skills needed to use technology.[12]

Urban school districts in California remained online throughout the 2020–21 academic year. By October 2020, local news media reported that, "Language barriers, limited computer skills, and long workdays outside the home have left many Latino immigrant parents frustrated by their own limitations and worried that with the school year already two months underway, their kids are falling behind."[13] One academic study of Latina mothers during the pandemic found that, "Their challenges included limited English proficiency when using online platforms and communicating with teachers, insufficient time at home, economic hardships, and increased mental health struggles for themselves and family members."[14] Researchers found that Latina mothers did all they could to assist their children. They had to learn in order for their children to learn. Many school districts offered virtual workshops in Spanish and other languages to help teach parents how to work Google Classroom, Zoom, and other resources children needed. However, in order to attend these workshops and supervise their children during online school hours, many Latina mothers had to switch to night shifts, significantly reduce their work hours, or quit their jobs.[15]

During this time, I unexpectedly became a computer tutor for other Latina moms as they struggled to support their kids with online learning. Before the pandemic, my tia, who immigrated from Mexico about fifteen years ago, worked sewing T-shirts in a garment factory. When the factory closed due to COVID-19, she lost her job and could not afford to pay for internet service.[16] Luckily, my sister who lives next door shared her Wi-Fi so that my tia's children, Lupita and Efren, ages ten and seven, could attend online school. My tia asked me to come over and help because they had never had a computer at home and did not know how to log onto the student portal to access the programs they needed for math and reading. In the early weeks of the pandemic, she and I put ourselves at risk of infection to see each other so that my young cousins could access online school. My tia's friend, another immigrant mother, also reached out for help. While the school was doing their best to assist her and her children, they needed additional hands-on computer instruction in Spanish.

Chromebooks, internet hotspots, and computer lessons from more experienced relatives and friends were not enough to prevent Latino students from falling behind academically during the pandemic. As academic support like after-school tutoring programs were canceled or kids were too burned out from sitting in front a screen all day to do more screen time with a tutor, all parents had to step in to supplement their children's education. Yet, even before COVID-19, many low-income immigrant parents struggled to help their children with homework because they did not speak English and had limited education.[17] Distance learning further disadvantaged immigrant parents from helping their children with computer and internet problems on top of academic work.[18]

Before the pandemic, my tia worked long hours and her children went to an afterschool program for supplemental tutoring. The lockdown period of the pandemic gave her time to focus on her children during the day; however, because she has only a primary school education, she was not equipped to act as an academic tutor and homework helper. She could only encourage her kids to learn on their own and sit with them while they were in online class to ensure they stayed focused. She despaired as her son missed online assignments and began falling behind in the second grade.

I could relate. I speak English fluently, am attending a four-year university, and have used a computer since the age of thirteen. And, still, I too was overwhelmed and anxious about how to best support my child in his remote schooling. Leo's excitement for "Zoom school" quickly wore off and we struggled. I would sometimes find him hiding under his desk because he couldn't understand his teacher or "the other kids won't stop talking and I can't hear anything." This gave me a lot of anxiety, as I did not want him to have a negative connection to school. I worried that when it came time to return to in-person learning, he would not want to or that he would fall behind in school because he frequently got very frustrated with online learning. There were many occasions when he would walk away or hide and I would hear his teacher call out "Leonardo . . . Leonardo, where did you go?" I had to walk away from my own online class session, or stop doing my homework, in order to talk to him so that he could sit back down and continue with school.

The COVID-19 pandemic intensified the educational disparities and technological divides that already stratified US society by social class, race, and citizenship status. Parents and children who were already struggling within the nation's educational system found themselves even more disadvantaged. Three years into the pandemic, there has been public alarm about how nonwhite students, low-income, and/or immigrant students fell behind academically as a result of school closures. By not talking about preexisting structural inequities, public discourse around this problem risks reinforcing racist and classist stereotypes of students of color as inherently less academically successful or motivated. In fact, long before the pandemic, government leaders and school administrators were aware that students of color—and entire low-income neighborhoods—faced a significant gap in technological access that put them at an academic disadvantage relative to their middle-class, white peers. Only after COVID-19 forced schools to close, and when low-income students were threatened with not being able to access school altogether, did school districts scramble to pass out second-rate computer devices and implement band-aid strategies to mitigate deeply entrenched technological inequities. Low-income students and their parents were expected to figure the rest out on their own, and when they could not, they were blamed and portrayed as academically deficient. Our children deserve better.

CHAPTER 24

Safer at Home? Negotiating Religion, UndocuLife, and Queerness During the COVID-19 Pandemic

Manuel (Manny) Ibarra

On March 19, 2020, Los Angeles Mayor Eric Garcetti announced the "Safer at Home Order for Control of COVID-19," which temporarily closed all but "essential" businesses and prohibited city residents from gathering with people from outside their household. The next day, Governor Gavin Newsom implemented a similar statewide order. "Safer at Home" would become the public motto of the pandemic, with closed schools and rolling lockdowns continuing through 2021. The purpose of these orders, according to the LA County Health Department's website, was to safeguard public safety and "protect the most vulnerable members of our community."[1] Residents were told that in order to stop the spread of the deadly virus, we should stay in our private homes where we would be shielded from harm. Public health officials and the news media called on Californians to retreat from the chaos of the pandemic into the safety and care of our homes.

But what if home is not a safe space? Chicana feminist sociologist Elisa Facio writes that, "Home can also be a site of disappointment, betrayal, violence, anguish, and uncertainty."[2] This reframing of home resonates with me as an undocumented and queer college student. Fear of deportation prevents me from attaching myself to a physical place that can be taken from me at any given point. Home is not a reliable refuge for undocumented people, since we can't tether to a country that has denied us access. I cannot root in soil that has been claimed by a capitalist white supremacist nation, even though my Mexican antepasados were here first in California. Nor is my nuclear family's home a source of safety because of my sexuality and gender expression. This space is unhealthy, toxic, and violent. It is quite the opposite of what a home is supposed to be. For the past two years I have been wondering, if undocuqueer youth are not "safer at home," where are we supposed to go during the pandemic?

My home has been in constant flux. Soon after I was born, my father migrated to "El Norte" in search of work, leaving me and my mother behind. As a six-year-old boy I endured the trauma of being torn away from a loving extended family in Mexico. Once in Los Angeles, I was thrust into an educational system that lacked the resources and knowledge to support migrant children with their transition to US society. Perhaps one of my most painful experiences as child was witnessing from a distance while my grandma was slowly taken by cancer, and not being able to visit her in Mexico before she died because my undocumented status in this country denies our human rights. At this moment I felt powerless. My grandma had been the matriarchal figure who glued our family together and loved me unconditionally. The racist laws of this country prevented from being with her in her final moments, further alienating me from this country that was to be my new home.

The last thing that shook my home life to the root foundation was my sexuality. I still remember my mother finding the strip of photo booth prints among all my other pictures that decorated my small bedroom. The photos were from one of my first dates when I was starting to explore my sexuality. It was my first year of college, and I was beginning to feel comfortable with myself. They were innocently sappy Valentine's photo-strips from the mall: four small square images, and in the last one, I was giving him a kiss on the cheek. As soon as my mom saw the photo-strip, she ripped it off the wall and crumbled it up. The first thing she asked was "Que va a decir tu papá?" I did not know what my father would say, but for a second, I felt courage. For a moment I had faith that our Jesus-filled home would become one of those cheesy coming-out stories on Latinx social media where the parents say, "We already knew, mijo. We love you no matter what." I couldn't have been more wrong.

My parents have been going to the same Catholic church for as long as I remember. Since migrating to the United States, they have been active in El Movimiento Familiar Cristiano Católico, a global evangelical organization run by the Catholic Church that promotes a "Christ-centered marriage" and "family values" through counseling, classes, and social activities for heterosexual couples and their children. My parents are now the presidents of a local chapter and oversee two parishes. They often spend more time at church meetings than at home.

When my parents found out I was queer, they waited until my younger sister was out of the house, held my hand, looked me in the eyes and told me I had a demon inside and needed to seek help. They told me that I was destroying the Christian family that they had put all their hard work into creating. As undocumented immigrants in the United States, they have struggled to achieve the hetero-patriarchal family standard, where my dad is the sole breadwinner and my mom is a stay-at-home wife. They have two polite and well-mannered children, who from a young age have impressed the church community with our maturity and responsibility. My sister and I were never kids who ran around making a mess at parties. We would be ashamed to, even for the slightest moment, step out of line. Since a young age we have been controlled. Under constant surveillance at home, we have been reminded how to talk, shake hands, eat, laugh. We are expected to be perfect and presentable, living proof that the Ibarras are the ideal Catholic Mexican family. I saw in my parents' eyes how my mere existence threatened the image they had carefully cultivated and projected to the world.

After my mother's discovery of the photos, I had to endure daily lectures during which I was not allowed to talk back. I was meant to sit and listen until I reached a breaking point and renounced my "sinful" behavior. I spoke up, and that is when I saw rage. I elected not to speak to my parents because of the hurt they caused but also to protect my physical self as I did not know what my anger-driven father would be capable of once he goes red. They stared at me, as though they could not recognize their son, as if they were confronting a stranger in their home.

Before the "Safer at Home" orders, I made it a point to never be at home. I would be busy either with my classes as a full-time student at Cal State LA or at work. Before I was old enough to have a work permit, I started working under the table, selling goods at the swapmeet, helping out at my uncle's party rental business, or with my dad at his machinist job. My first "legal" job after I got a work permit through DACA was at Jersey Mike's. I was hired on my eighteenth birthday and two years later, I picked up a second job at Chipotle. Both of these jobs were supposed to be part-time, but because I was part of the management team at both stores, this was unrealistic. I was constantly on call and usually ended up working more than forty hours per week, but only received the benefits of a part-time worker. My weekdays involved waking up at 5 a.m. to make it to my first class at 7. After classes, I would go straight to work and would not get home until 11 p.m., when I would finally have time to focus on homework as late into the night as my body would let me. Then I repeated the same routine over again the next day. It was a hectic cycle but one that allowed me to be out of danger of being home while my parents were awake. After I had told them about my sexuality and we had ruptured our relationship, being out of the house during the day prevented altercations and gave me a sense of security. Avoidance was my strategy to protect myself and prevent any arguments over my sexuality.

When the pandemic hit, I was forced to do online schooling while trapped at home. My parents rent a tiny house in a working-middle-class Latino and Asian suburb of the San Gabriel Valley. When we first moved in, the space we rented included one bedroom, one bathroom, a small kitchen, and a living room. My mom, dad, and sister shared the bedroom, and I slept in the living room on an old sofa that caused me back problems. (The subject of constant family conversation where my mom would say she wants to get rid of the couch, which has been patched up many times, yet she knows replacing it is out of our budget.) We lived like that for eight years until the landlord's nephew moved out from the small room that was connected to the kitchen, and I moved into that tight space which could fit only a twin bed and desk. My new room did not have a door. That meant zero privacy, being watched and having to perform hetero-masculinity 24/7.

I remember being in online class and stepping into the kitchen to get a glass of water. It was a hot day and the A/C stopped working, so I had my hair tied up in a ponytail away from my face. I did not know my dad had come home early from work, and at the sight of my hair he lost his temper because "no real man has long hair" and "would dare to wear such a feminine style." The situation escalated to the point where my mom was begging me to let my hair down, while trying to physically restrain my dad. I had to get out of the house because, although I was trying to conceal my fear and stand up for myself, I knew that I was not safe. I logged out of class and drove to my friend's house where I just laid in her bed and felt relief being away from home. By nightfall I had to return to face my parents. While I wanted to leave home and escape permanently, realistically I had no safe space to run to.

Since the start of the pandemic, LGBTQ+ advocates have challenged the "safer at home" ideology by highlighting the stigma, alienation, and violence that many queer and trans people face in their home spaces. This is especially true for LGBTQ+ youth, who suffer the highest suicide and homelessness rates among their peers, due to homophobic and transphobic rejection and violence from family members. One study of students across 254 colleges found that "nearly half (45.7%) of LGBT college students have immediate families that do not support or know their LGBT identity. Approximately 60% of sampled LGBT college students were experiencing psychological distress, anxiety, and depression during the pandemic as a result of having to move back home.[3] Another study by the UCLA Williams Institute found that LGBTQ+ college students were almost twice as likely as non-LGBTQ+ students to experience a housing disruption due to the pandemic, including being forced out of student housing and having to move into their own apartment or shared housing with others.[4]

Just as COVID-19 altered my personal safety protocols, the pandemic and the government's response to it also weakened the systems that undocumented students and our families have developed to navigate the structural violence that we encounter. A 2021 study of undocumented college students in California found that, "The vast majority . . . acknowledged that federal policies prevented undocumented immigrants, and their citizen family members, from accessing economic relief provided by the March 2020 Coronavirus Aid, Relief, and Economic Security (CARES) Act."[5] The State of California created a $125 million disaster relief fund for working undocumented Californians who were impacted by COVID-19 and whose immigration status made them ineligible for unemployment insurance benefits and CARES Act benefits. This fund distributed a one-time payment of $500 per adult, with a cap of $1,000 per household, to one hundred fifty thousand undocumented workers (a small fraction of the two million undocumented people in California). However, my dad did not receive any help from federal or state COVID relief packages. Although he has been working as a machinist for the same company for two decades, he receives no sick days, paid vacation, overtime, or other employment-based benefits. As an "essential worker," he did not have the option to stop working during the lockdown phase of the pandemic. Similarly, many other undocumented college students reported that their family members were "essential workers" in workplaces that did not maintain strict COVID safety protocols or offer paid medical leave.[6]

The pandemic forced undocumented queer Latinx youth, like me, to endure being trapped in unsafe spaces. During the first sixteen months of the pandemic, my relationship with my parents was the worst it had ever been because I had no option but to stay home in the toxic environment. In August 2021, I was hired as a residential assistant in the university dorms where I lived with and supported other LGBTQ+ students of color. Finally, I was able to create my own safe space and haven away from toxicity. Living away from my family in the dorms gave me the privilege of redefining "home" on my own terms and expressing my authentic self in a safe and nurturing environment—something that is not possible for many other undocumented queer individuals.

Queer undocumented Latinx youth continue to struggle to define "home" as we navigate multiple intersecting borderlands, or heridas, as Gloria Anzaldua calls them.[7] These heridas (wounds) slowly cut to our core, jabs from immigration laws, exploitation of our people, homophobia within our culture. We experience a constant cutting into our identity, as US society and our families try to force us into a perfect mold of acceptability. Yet we remain standing while wounded. We remain embraced with our own joteria (queer Latinx) community that nourishes and protects our spirit.[8]

Author's Note

While writing this essay, I struggled with focusing on negative aspects of my testimonio, especially on challenging family dynamics. As children of immigrants and first-generation college students, we tend to focus on our parents' sacrifice and resilience because we see firsthand how this country degrades and exploits brown immigrant bodies. For as long as I've been in the United States, I have focused on shielding my parents from harm, making it difficult to express my true identity and how my parents' controlling behavior and rejection of my queerness have damaged me. I want to honor the love and guidance mis padres have given me, yet also acknowledge the challenges in our relationship. I chose to write about these family fractures and share my experience in its true form in order to support my healing journey and help those who have similar experiences. I love my parents—los amo—and am forever grateful to them, but now am learning to heal.

CHAPTER 25

Autoethnographies from the "Sacrifice Zone" of Latinx Los Angeles

Alejandra Marchevsky

April 2020: The squares slowly populate with students' faces. They log in from Boyle Heights, Watts, South Gate, Montebello, and as far as Orange County. Class starts at 6 p.m., peak activity time in students' tight living quarters. Most Zoom from their kitchen table, so we can see their parents, spouses, children, and siblings cooking and folding laundry in the background. In a twist on California car culture, several join from smartphones in their parked vehicle, where they can participate in class without relatives or roommates listening in. One student logs in from inside her bedroom closet, the only place that affords concentration and privacy.

Magaly opens tonight's well-being check-in. She sits so close to her laptop that I can see red welts from the face mask she wore during her ten-hour work shift. Magaly's job at McDonald's is her family's only source of income.[1] Her parents lost their jobs due to the coronavirus, and relief benefits are unavailable because they are undocumented. Seven people crowd into a two-bedroom house in South LA. Every space in Magaly's life feels tight. Even though the dining room of McDonald's is like a ghost town, the back of the restaurant is cramped with workers. Her boss received a federal COVID-19 small business grant that requires that a majority of his employees work every day. At a time when the public is exhorted to socially distance, Magaly and her Latinx and African American coworkers must stand shoulder to shoulder in a hot industrial kitchen, suffocating in double-layered surgical masks and praying they don't bring the deadly virus home.

Jasmine speaks next on the theme of female sacrificio. Californians have been ordered to "shelter-in-place," yet her mother goes out every day to work in the homes of wealthy white people. One employer is a Trump supporter who forbids her to wear a protective mask while she cleans the house. The public celebrates workers like her mom as pandemic heroes, but she has no other choice. She is the only family member left with work, and their savings are rapidly depleting. Last semester, Jasmine commuted thirty miles every day to attend college, and her part-time job helped pay her family's rent. Now, with her workplace and campus shuttered, Jasmine does all the domestic labor at home: cooking for five people, washing dishes and laundry, overseeing her younger siblings' online schooling, and consoling them through this traumatic time. This is her responsibility as the eldest daughter in a Mexican immigrant family. Jasmine theorizes eloquently about how the pandemic has intensified the sacrifice expected of Latinas as disposable domestics for US society and care workers for their own families and communities.

Comments stream into the chat field as Jasmine and Magaly speak:

"You got this, mujer! No te desesperes"
"We are here for you."
"Fuck racial capitalism!"
"El machismo apesta!"

Our feminista online learning community is a lifeboat we cling to.

Autoethnography in "Tight Spaces"

The essays in this section were written by students in my women's, gender, and sexuality studies classes at California State University, Los Angeles, a regional public university that serves a majority population of first-generation students of color. Located in East Los Angeles—a hub of Mexican American life in the city—Cal State L.A. ranks fifth nationally among four-year colleges with the highest percentage of Latinx students.[2] Most Cal State L.A. students rely on financial aid and low-wage work to meet their basic needs, live with their families, and regularly skip meals and medical care because they cannot afford them.

Over twenty years of teaching at Cal State L.A., I have grappled with how race and class differences place me in a "fixed relation" (using poet June

Jordan's words) to my students.[3] As an Argentinian immigrant who grew up in the United States, I connect with Mexican and Central American students around shared cultural references and experiences navigating between our home cultures and Anglo-American society. With Latina students, we bond over our resistance to the gender expectations of "dutiful daughters" and "mujeres decentes" in our Latin American cultures. However, it has always been clear that the privileges that US society confers on me based on whiteness, class, and citizenship protect me from the structural racism that plagues Cal State LA students' lives.

The COVID-19 crisis exponentially heightened the imbalance of vulnerability between me and my students. Like most affluent Californians, my family weathered the worst period of the pandemic from our comfortable home, telecommuting to work, with groceries and take-out food delivered, and accessing quality (if strained) telehealth services. We despaired over the collective crisis, feared catching the virus, grumbled about being shut in together, and listened to our teenage son complain that he missed his friends and hated online school—but our material needs were never imperiled. Meanwhile, precarity spiraled among Cal State L.A. students: unemployment, poverty, unstable housing, medical apartheid, violence, digital inequality, repressive immigration laws, and racialized policing. As students' communities became COVID-19 epicenters in LA. County, the cruel gap between their life conditions and mine widened. It was a tale of two pandemics.

Cal State L.A. students activated rich family and community care networks for pandemic survival. They planted community gardens, cared for children and elderly relatives, helped relatives and neighbors access COVID-19 testing and vaccination websites, organized ride sharing, and volunteered with mutual-aid projects. These activities pointed to the failure of US society to meet the structural crisis and the need for collective solutions. Yet, by the second year of the pandemic, the government response had shifted to making individuals primarily responsible for managing viral risk. The media framed disproportionately high infection and death rates among people of color as epidemiologically determined—by preexisting medical conditions and "high-risk" social settings—rather than as socioeconomically produced. I grew increasingly alarmed by how these ideas were creeping into my online classroom. Whereas students previously shared openly when they were infected with the virus, this information was now whispered during office hours. Class discussions in the spring semester of 2020 voiced collective anger about unsafe working conditions and long waitlists for campus psychological services. A year later, the structure of feeling among students had shifted to resignation and grit. Sickness, food and cash scarcity, houselessness, unstable Wi-Fi service, and dropping grades increasingly boomeranged back to students as their fault and responsibility.

I had been following the pandemic autoethnography project led by my close friend Jeanne Theoharis and her colleagues at Brooklyn College. When essays by Brooklyn College students were published by *Black Perspectives*, I was transfixed. The embodied knowledge and sociopolitical framing in these students' writing surpassed most journalistic and scholarly accounts of social inequality and the pandemic. The student authors from New York City sounded like my students in Los Angeles. These essays convinced me of the power of autoethnography as a methodology through which my students could research from their social location and turn their pandemic experiences outward to critical analysis and political critique.[4] I began offering an autoethnographic assignment in my courses where students could document and analyze their personal experience using our class texts and additional research.

Students created a range of autoethnographies on topics as diverse as housing insecurity among trans people, gun violence, gender-affirming medical care, sexual privacy and autonomy, revolutionary queer mothering, and immigrant women and street vending. Some were later invited to commit to regular meetings with me, additional research, and multiple revisions and drafts of their essays for inclusion in this book. Because of the commitment this required, and the immense stress they were facing, only four students— all first-generation students of Mexican heritage—were able to work closely with me for an additional year to revise their work.

These essays were written from what Chicana theorist Cindy Cruz calls the "tight spaces" where queer, trans, and femme Latinx youth live.[5] Two of the authors are women and two are nonbinary queer folks. One is a mother with young children, and another is a person with disabilities. At least one is formerly undocumented, and three have parents or other relatives who are undocumented. All are low-wage workers in their twenties who live with their nuclear or extended families, and whose paychecks are essential for their family to meet its basic needs. These students sacrificed scarce personal time to do the intellectual labor for this book, and having to delve into traumatic experiences and subjects took a toll on their emotional well-being.

They persisted because they saw the power of "researching back," which Maori scholar Linda Tuhiwai Smith describes as a process through which indigenous and other marginalized communities engage in "a recovery of ourselves, an analysis of colonialism, and a struggle for self-determination."[6] Over and over, these students told me this autoethnography project was a way to "give back" to their community through counter-storytelling that centered communal knowledges and perspectives that would otherwise be left out of the public accounts of COVID-19. Far surpassing what I could imagine at the outset of this project, students seized on autoethnography as a means to, in the words of feminist philosopher Maria Lugones, witness and write publicly "against the grain of power."[7]

Structuring Latinx Lives in LA's "Sacrifice Zone"

Historian Julie Livingston observes that, even before the COVID-19 crisis, the United States "had already honed a sacrifice zone—the place just offstage, obscured from view, where the well-being of some is seized as an offering toward some higher purpose called 'the economy.'"[8] During the pandemic, a generation of working-class Latinx fathers and mothers, siblings and cousins has been sacrificed so that other Angelenos can buy fresh produce, order take-out, work from home while their children are cared for, and have their houses cleaned. In documenting and critically framing these stories, the autoethnographies from Latinx LA move the "sacrifice zone" from "just off-stage" into unforgiving public view.

In truth, Latinx people lived in this sacrifice zone well before 2020. Throughout US history, Latinx workers have been economically indispensable, yet treated as dispensable, relegated to low-paying jobs where they risk injury and disease, and threatened with deportation when they claim basic rights. COVID-19 drove this hyper-exploitation of Latinx labor to an unprecedented scale. Concentrated in front-line occupations in domestic services, agriculture, meat packing, health care, construction, and restaurants, immigrants from Mexico and Central America and many of their US-born children and grandchildren kept our economy running during the pandemic. Most worked in jobs that could not be done remotely in crowded workplaces with poor ventilation, and for employers who do not provide PPE, sick pay, or health insurance.[9] The human cost has been immeasurable, especially in

Los Angeles. Latinx people comprise half of LA County residents, yet *by far* the greatest number of COVID-19 infections and deaths. In August 2022 (when the County still reliably tracked COVID numbers), Latinx residents accounted for over 1.3 million COVID-19 cases, followed at a distant second by white residents at less than half a million cases.[10] Latinx deaths, for any cause, jumped by 48% from 2020 to 2022—an unprecedented leap that experts attribute to higher rates of exposure and health risk due to lack of access to quality medical care and higher prevalence of comorbidities like hypertension, diabetes, and lung disease.[11]

While national media coverage and public health data have highlighted the pandemic's disproportionate harm to Latinx people, this problem has been largely cast as tragic but inevitable—in the glib words of one news report on East LA, "a perfect storm" that befell Latinx communities.[12] The pandemic autoethnographies by Cal State LA students challenge this pervasive view of Latinx people as "naturally" vulnerable. The authors combine firsthand accounts of their experiences with empirical data about low-wage jobs, unhealthy and unsafe workplaces, wage theft, and segregated neighborhoods, workplaces, and schools, to present a complex account of how Latinx people are *made vulnerable* by racial capitalism, anti-immigrant policies, and the neoliberal dismantling of public services. These autoethnographies unsettle and complicate explanations that entered our collective consciousness in 2020—"essential worker," "preexisting conditions," "safer at home," and "vulnerable communities." They teach us how structural inequity created the pandemic crisis for LA's Latinx working-class residents, a scene that would repeat across the nation for Latinx communities in Texas, Georgia, New York, Michigan, Oregon, and Alabama.[13]

Though topically diverse, these autoethnographies all examine the ways that family—biological and chosen—saved Latinx communities when neither the labor market nor the state provided for their basic needs. In these essays, we see children and grandchildren taking care of grandparents, young people providing critical health care to sick family members, friends offering safe shelter from violence, elders doing childcare, circles of sisters and tias collaborating to ensure that youth have access to schooling, and college students working more hours than ever to provide for their family's economic needs. Today, several years into the pandemic, Latinx families are still strained beyond their limits as they struggle to compensate for the essential rights that would be available in a healthy democracy: strong labor laws that protect workers from wage exploitation and unsafe working conditions, a system of accessible and quality health care, a social welfare system that adequately provides for elders and low-income families, and well-funded and equitable public K–12 and higher education systems.

Yet, the Cal State LA student authors reject an uncritical celebration of "familismo" in Latinx culture, or moralistic and neoliberal parables of immigrant families helping themselves in the hardest of times. Instead, drawing on intersectional feminist and queer frameworks, they present a complex look at Latinx families as structured in uneven power, exploitation, and violence. They write bravely about how homophobia and transphobia in Latinx families made home for LGBTQ Latinx college students a more dangerous space during the "shelter-at-home" stage of the pandemic. Machismo is shown to be harmful to children and families, but also victimizes working fathers, whose culturally situated identities as fearless men and responsible providers propel them into unsafe workplaces, where they are exposed to the virus, illness and death. These autoethnographies urgently remind us that, when the state underfunds or dismantles crucial public services, it falls on women of color and LGBTQ people of color to take responsibility for the undervalued gendered care that shoulders the survival of communities of color.

Mapping Segregation and Latinx COVID "Hot Spots" in LA

In the LA autoethnographies, racial segregation is a salient backdrop for the stories that students tell and problems they research. The essays document social worlds where the authors share workplaces, housing, schools, churches, and public transit almost exclusively with other people of color, most of them Latinx. Wendy Casillas describes their grandparents' modest home in the only corner of the San Fernando Valley where Mexicans were allowed to purchase property in the first half of the twentieth century and today is still home to a majority of Mexican and other Latinx people. Maria Cerezo and Manny Ibarra's fathers worked in construction sites and machinist shops exclusively with other Latino immigrant men where the virus spread due to a lack of health safety measures.

While journalists and scholars have devoted much attention to racial disparities surrounding COVID-19, they have largely overlooked the role of racial and class segregation in producing epidemiological inequality.[14] Of the ten most segregated areas in California, seven are Latinx-majority areas located in LA County. East LA, where Cal State LA is located, ranks #1 on this list.[15] Latinx residents are also most likely to be concentrated in brown-collar jobs in light manufacturing, service jobs, and agriculture and food processing, where they work primarily with people of the same ethnicity. These patterns of segregation do not reflect individual preferences for jobs or neighborhoods, but rather have been engineered over decades by racist hiring practices and discriminatory zoning, lending, and real estate practices by white politicians, housing developers, banks, and homeowners. Los Angeles's planned segregation manifests as COVID-19 hot spots, and partially explains the virus's spread among Latinx residents, who are most likely to be infected and unknowingly pass it on to each other in work and neighborhood spaces.

In the first summer of the pandemic, COVID-19 infections grew by over 1,000% in areas where the majority of residents are Latinx, like Southeast LA, where Manny grew up. By March 2021, Latinx neighborhoods had infection rates of nearly three times as many cases as areas with low numbers of Latinx residents. Wendy's frail grandfather could not go outside because their community had one of the highest COVID rates in the nation.[16] These narratives force us to examine why these Latinx communities continued to be viral hot spots as the pandemic marched on, whereas mortality and infection rates declined in whiter and more affluent communities.

On Heteropatriarchy and Latino Fathers as "Essential Workers"

Most explanations of the disproportionate number of Latinx infections and deaths from COVID-19 naturalize the concentration of Latinx workers who have been employed in high-risk workplaces throughout the pandemic. Echoing past historical archetypes—in particular the mid-twentieth-century Mexican "Bracero" worker—the pandemic introduced the image of the Latinx "essential worker" whose unquestioned economic subordination is cast in terms of self-gain (migrants grateful to earn dollars) and also in service to US national security in a moment of crisis. The autoethnographies from LA tackle head-on the hyper-exploitation of Latinx immigrant workers and

the public discourses and government practices that make this system possible. Their research and storytelling challenge the controlling image of Latinx
immigrant workers "who are happy to do the jobs that citizens don't want to
do." Manny's autoethnography interrupts this ideology by showing their father
was *not* an "essential worker" but "did not have the option to stop working
because his employer stayed open in violation of LA County health rules." This
was a common phenomenon in Los Angeles during the COVID-19 lockdown:
restaurants, upholstery shops, car washes—industries that rely on undocumented workers—opened in defiance of public health rules. City leaders
threatened businesses who stayed open during the lockdown with hefty fines,
but in reality, enforcement was spotty. Manny shows how employers violated
the law, the government failed to enforce immigrant workers' rights, and
unlike more privileged workers who could telecommute or were eligible to
receive unemployment and COVID-19 relief, undocumented workers faced
an impossible choice between starvation or unsafe work.

Similarly, Maria's essay refuses to see her father's death from COVID-19
as explained by a vague vulnerability that society now associates with "essential" workers, especially those who are undocumented. She first questions
how certain work was politically constructed as "essential," revealing that
LA Mayor Eric Garcetti's decision to classify construction as an "essential
industry" was a concession to the powerful construction lobby. Moreover,
although city rules required that construction sites enforce social distancing between workers and provide hand washing stations and PPE, Maria
documents how Latino immigrants were *made* vulnerable to COVID-19
by the lack of government inspections at construction sites even before the
pandemic. Her analysis also illuminates how Latino immigrant men may
"consent" to and perpetuate unsafe working conditions—such as not wearing a mask or social distancing—due to coercive brown collar workplace
cultures and cultural norms that associate masculinity and fatherhood with
taking risks to provide for your family's needs. Ultimately, the ability of the
construction industry to continue to operate without increased safety costs
and labor disruptions during the pandemic benefited both employers' and
consumers' bottom lines.

Furthermore, while much research on racial disparities in preexisting
health conditions and COVID illness has emphasized poor people's and
people of color's lack of access to preventive medical care, Maria directs our

attention to toxic workplaces as directly responsible for COVID-19 deaths. Her research traces her father's severe COVID-19 illness to the construction industry where toxic contaminants ravage workers' lungs, and where employers, industry lobbyists and government regulators have been aware of these workplace dangers but have failed to protect workers. Airborne particles and contaminants pervade industries where Latinx immigrant workers are concentrated: construction sites, light and labor-intensive manufacturing, and trucking and industrial transportation. Harmful chemicals follow Latinx workers home in LA County, where they are more likely to live near toxic sites than their ethnic counterparts in any other US city.[17]

When read together, Manny's and Maria's autoethnographies powerfully situate Latinx workers in a matrix of exploitative and dangerous employer practices bolstered by a lack of government regulations to protect workers. Maria's "social forensic" investigation of her father's death underscores how bodies of color are made vulnerable to COVID-19. These deaths and illnesses are not inevitable, but rather are caused by capitalist and state practices that fetishize economic growth and profit over human life.

Women and Queer Folks Doing "State Work"

In this book's introduction, Entin and Theoharis describe an "organized state abandonment" of low-income communities that went into overdrive during the pandemic. This theme runs through the autoethnographies from Latinx L.A. Elizabeth's son's public elementary school sits in central Long Beach, where nearly all of the students are low-income Latinxs, African Americans or Southeast Asians; across the city at the upscale Naples Elementary, about half the students are white and only a quarter economically disadvantaged. When her son's school distributes devices to students so they can log in to class from home, Elizabeth initially is relieved that the state has not abandoned her kindergartner and their community. That promise of equitable public education collapses in the chaos of old Chromebooks that don't work, teachers being thrust into remote teaching with inadequate support, and low-income students struggling to learn while they are constantly being "dropped" from online class meetings. In wealthy California—which, in 2021, generated a historic $300 billion tax surplus yet still ranked thirty-sixth in the nation in K–12 spending[18]—immigrant mothers struggle to ameliorate structural inequities so that their children can access quality education during the pandemic.[19] Similarly, Wendy's essay exposes not only their exploitation as a paid elderly caregiver, but also the state's refusal to invest in the care that elderly Mexican immigrants like their grandfather need and deserve. Like the broken laptops distributed to students at John Muir Elementary, California's IHSS program gestures toward equitable access to home care for low-income elderly Californians but falls far short.

Feminists have long argued that the neoliberal dismantling of social welfare systems across the world has depended on women's, and especially women of color's, hyper-exploited and often unpaid care work. Writing in the 1990s, M. Jacqui Alexander presciently observed that, as the state cuts "sectors which have been historically coded as women's work: health, clinic and hospital service, caring for the sick and elderly, social services and education . . . [it] relies upon and operates within these dominant constructions of a servile femininity, perennially willing and able to serve, a femininity that can automatically fill the gaps left by the state."[20] Indeed, when the state social worker approves *only four* hours apiece of daily home assistance for their infirm grandfather, Wendy and their uncle step up to provide unpaid round-the-clock care—exactly as the system is intended to work. This "choice" to work for free stems from a lack of another option, as well as by Latinx cultural expectations that Wendy, who is queer and nonbinary but was assigned female at birth and unmarried with no children, do the feminized work of elderly caregiving. Wendy's uncle, a bachelor and person with disabilities who shares the house with his father, also is assigned a feminized or queer status in the family through which his care work is also expected and exploited both by his family and the state. Similarly, Elizabeth and the other Latina moms in her network must mobilize to ensure that their children have full access to education during the pandemic. Sharing internet service so their kids can log in to class, risking infection to teach each other how to use a computer and navigate Zoom, sitting with their children throughout the school day to make sure they stay focused and the internet connection doesn't drop—these Latina mothers' unpaid cognitive labor was essential to the continuation of public schooling during more than a year when schools were physically closed in LA County. These autoethnographies show us women and queer people doing invisibilized state-work that was essential for their families, and also the LA region, to survive the pandemic.

Not "Safer at Home:" State Violence
Meets Family Violence

Families are spaces where Latinx people can nurture each other's well-being within a larger context of racist and neoliberal state abandonment. They can simultaneously be spaces of harm, where family members exploit, control, denigrate or violate each other. Manny's essay sheds light on how public and private violence intensified in the lives of undocuqueer youth during the pandemic. For Manny, whose sexuality cannot be spoken or seen at home, writing is an act of self-naming and self-determination. Their essay powerfully argues that "safer at home" rested on a hetero-patriarchal, middle-class, and citizen-centered ideal of the home. Manny reminds us that because ICE can enter a private family home and expel migrants from the country, many undocumented people have difficulty laying down settled roots in the United States (especially as the first year of the pandemic overlapped with arguably the most anti-immigrant White House and Congress in US history). Manny's simultaneous account of the intensified surveillance and homophobia they endured from their parents sheds light on the threats to the safety and mental health of LGBTQ students during the pandemic. Media and scholarly attention to this problem has been limited to students at residential colleges. Wendy's autoethnography also speaks to the violence of cis-heteronormativity in Latinx families, as they write about their grandfather's increasingly inappropriate sexual attention, his mis-gendering of them, and pressure to fit a heterosexual and cisgender norm. For Wendy, autoethnographic writing enabled a new self-understanding as a gender nonbinary family care worker within a patriarchal capitalist system, deconstructing family ideologies and expectations around elder care through a feminist and queer lens.

Manny and Wendy's essays demonstrate that factors of social vulnerability—racism, poverty, immigration status, housing insecurity, unemployment or underemployment, etc.—intersected with gender and sexuality to make some LGBTQ college students more vulnerable to gender-based victimization and violence at home during the COVID-19 pandemic.[21] They beautifully document the "sacrifice zone" that queer Latinx people are expected to live within their families. Through their research and writing, these students refuse to sacrifice their own gender and sexual self-definitions as an offering to a "higher ideal" that is la familia.

"Femmes and Queers of Color to the Front"

In moments of crisis across history, the concerns of women and LGBTQ people have been silenced and marginalized by those who insist we must focus on more pressing problems, like economic survival and racial inequality; matters of gender and sexual inequity must wait to be addressed in less urgent times. This ideology pervades public responses to COVID-19, where data on women's and LGBTQ people's vulnerability to the virus has received far less attention. Public concerns about women's health during the pandemic has been tellingly focused on the virus's effect on fetal health (because women's bodies are only seen as vessels for reproduction). In the first year of the pandemic, shelter-at-home policies and school closures animated public discussion about the gendered division of household labor and its inequitable consequences for women's labor and well-being. Yet most public framings of this issue perpetuated a middle-class white feminist narrative that centered heterosexual women in professional careers who struggled to telecommute to work during the lock-down phase of the pandemic while meeting their family's increased demands for childcare, cooking, laundry, and housecleaning. Poor women, trans women, Black women, immigrant women, nonbinary folks, and queer men of color were simply expected to continue as before, exposing our society's reliance on and extreme degradation of feminized care work.

By bringing "femmes and queers of color to the front," the Cal State L.A. autoethnographies demonstrate the need for intersectional frameworks for understanding and developing responses to the ongoing global crisis of COVID-19. The essays provide a complex understanding of gendered family care in working-class communities of color, demonstrating that while the responsibility for families' physical and emotional survival falls heavily on mothers, it also pulls in daughters, abuelas and tias, gay men, and other queer folks. In my two decades of teaching before the pandemic, I witnessed tens of dozens of Latinx women, nonbinary students, and queer male students struggle to balance school with extraordinary family responsibilities. This labor is expected and exploited due to patriarchal ideologies and social structures that are perpetuated in private households and public institutions alike. Through their family care work before the pandemic—which often also extended to volunteer service in their communities—these young people were making up for the lack of universal health care and childcare, underfunded public transit systems and urban public schools, and government institutions and actors that are hostile or indifferent to people of color and immigrants. After 2020, when Latinx communities were under siege and the state offered very little support, these same working-class Latina and Latinx students became essential caregivers on myriad levels that have not yet been recognized or valued by our society.

"Defining Ourselves for Ourselves"

> For Black women as well as Black men, it is axiomatic that if we do not define ourselves for ourselves, we will be defined by others—for their use, and to our detriment.
> —Audre Lorde, *Sister Outsider*

> Our voices are our weapons, they have the power to shatter the systems that keep us oppressed."
> —Cherrie Moraga

Finally, amid public proclamations that the pandemic is over and normal life is back, these autoethnographies underscore that this is not true for Latinx Angelinos. In LA County today Latinx residents continue to have the highest COVID-19 infection and mortality rates. The percentage of Latinx people in LA's unhoused population has grown significantly over the past two years. As the crisis continues, these autoethnographic narratives interrupt public nostalgia for "normal life." They document a toxic normal that existed for Latinx communities long before 2020, and that was contorted into newly deadly and destabilizing forms after the arrival of the virus to Los Angeles. For Maria, that toxic normal included the known pollutants that damaged her father's lungs, as well as the damaging patriarchal norms that discourage immigrant men from complaining about unsafe working conditions, due to fear of being cast as unmanly or getting fired for being too difficult. For Wendy, a return to pre-2020—which they describe as a time when they were "living my best life"—involved working two poverty-wage jobs to be able to afford rent, food, and a public education.

These young Latinx scholars challenge and inspire us to imagine and build a more humane and radically just normal. Their pieces reveal how the vocabulary that emerged to frame and understand the pandemic—"shelter at home," "essential workers," "safer at home," "preexisting conditions"—erased the realities of many of the hardest-hit communities, and was deployed to their profound detriment. As Toni Morrison writes, "Definitions always belong to the definers, not the defined." These pieces flip the lens. They reveal a more accurate language for understanding the pandemic—socially manufactured vulnerability, sacrifice zones, premature death, essential-but-disposable workers.

But knowing that, reading that, is not enough. For readers on the other side of the sacrifice zone, the pieces in this book call us to be co-conspirators. The authors demand of us what Lugones calls "faithful witnessing."[22] This involves scholars and policy makers aligning with oppressed communities, centering them not only as storytellers but as community scholars who advance vital understandings of systems of injustice. The essays in this book demonstrate how the self-definitions and analyses produced from students in the "sacrifice zone" challenge the dominant framing of the COVID-19 pandemic. "Faithful witnessing" calls on us, as readers, to deploy our privilege—even at risk of our institutional stature or material and political safety—to act in solidarity with these students and their communities to transform these systems of cruel inequality.

Conclusion: This Book Is Not
a Conclusion to the Pandemic

Joseph Entin, Jeanne Theoharis, and Student Contributors

It's summer 2023 and, despite President Biden's declaration that the pandemic is over, it rolls on. Mask mandates have been lifted in public spaces, on airplanes, public schools, and doctors' offices, but hundreds of people are still dying each day from COVID in the United States. Medical researchers have not identified definitive causes or cures for long COVID. In New York, Mayor Eric Adams has ended the vaccine mandate for private employers, closed the city-run vaccination and testing sites, and proposed $200 million in cuts to the public school budget. Yet anyone who comes into contact with President Biden is still tested and air filtration has been improved—so the most powerful continue to have protections while the rest of the country is on its own. Inflation is spiking as corporations continue to generate massive profits. Reeling from the hardships of the pandemic, spiraling inequality, and the rapidly rising cost of rent and groceries, workers at Starbucks, Amazon, Trader Joe's and other companies have launched nationwide unionization campaigns—and Teamsters who work for UPS just averted a strike, winning substantial gains in the process.

In the first months of the pandemic, with rising consciousness of economic inequality, health precarity, and community vulnerability, there was a growing sense that the United States could *not* go back to the old normal—that we would have to forge things anew. The pandemic exposed a host of structural fault lines that rendered millions of people—especially, but by no means only, poor and working-class people, immigrants, communities of color—vulnerable to the cascading array of health, economic, and social problems that accompanied the coronavirus. It became clear that prevailing policies and patterns had to be revised to make American and world society more humane and more just.

That has certainly not happened . . . yet.

But it is that sense of urgent possibility—the belief that this doesn't have to be the way our society functions—that ripples through this project. These autoethnographies constitute an archive of what happened to families and communities in New York and Los Angeles, a historical record of what transpired for communities often left out of public storytelling. These pieces represent a refusal to be invisible, to go silently into the night. They tell truths that society has yet to reckon with.

But they are not simply a chronicle of pandemic experiences. More than that, these autoethnographies are a conduit to new ways of thinking and acting. The conviction that the perspectives included here can help reimagine our society propelled this project from a small summer grant initiative to this book.

Seen together, these student writings demand bigger reflection and a different kind of truth telling. They ask us to consider broad questions about how our world might be restructured: *What kind of society do we need to create going forward? How do we expose the fables our country tells itself about the pandemic and its ongoing impacts? How can we imagine a different normal— and what kinds of new thinking, new ways of organizing, and new policies could make this a better world?*

While ideas for transforming the ways society operates pop up across the pieces of the book, we convened most of the authors on Zoom in October 2022 to figure out the central ideas for the conclusion together. It was a way to confront the ongoing, kaleidoscopic impacts of the pandemic and to imagine collectively the society that we—the student writers and us—wanted and that our families and communities' well-being required.[1] What follows are some reflections and ideas for new directions, policies, and ways of relating to one another that emerged from our conversation and the students' pieces more generally. It is a call to reconsider, analyze, criticize, and most importantly act.

Our conversation began with the urgency of the project itself, as the writers underlined the importance of voicing stories for many people who have not had their experiences widely recognized. These pieces were painfully hard to write and rewrite, the authors attested, but we composed them to make experiences visible that are often invisibilized. We told a set of truths about the pandemic that this society was already trying to bury, the writers insisted. We wanted to show people they are not alone in these experiences and to testify to many avenues of inequality often ignored, in the hopes that things could change.

When we are seen, the authors in this book insist, the myths the United States tells itself about equality and opportunity and the pandemic being over begin to crumble. *When we are seen*, people who are dying, who are getting sick, who are being exploited for other people's comfort and wealth, are recognized. *When we are seen*, things cannot stay as they are. *When we are seen*, the student contributors make clear, the ease with which our society seeks to go back to "normal" is recognized as normalizing inequality and suffering.

These writings hold up the fractured mirror that is American society, and readers may not always like what they see: how this country, how racial capitalism, has operated and continues to operate in harmful and cruel ways that treat many lives as disposable. Other people's safety and security were protected by the ways our families' and community's lives were deemed less important, the student authors observed. These pieces reveal truths about the deep inequalities built into American society, politics, and economics, by exposing how all too often, people and communities without means or power are perversely held responsible for the problems they face. We are expected to be resilient, the contributors explained, to simply push past the barriers our society has set up. So much of the celebration of essential workers, offered by people whose work did not put them in jeopardy, was self-serving—pretty words rather than the real material acknowledgment (hazard pay, sick days, raises, universal access to health) we needed and deserved. No one wants to put their health at risk for their job. No one wants to have to be resilient.

What helped us survive the pandemic, our authors noted, was thinking and acting in ways that foregrounded community over individualism, brothers and sisters on the job, neighbors and the community we cherished and worked to protect. The pandemic demonstrated our interdependency—in our apartment buildings and neighborhoods, in our jobs, in our cities, in our world. It highlighted connections to people who are not immediately next to us and bonds to people farther away.

Yet Americans are often loath to acknowledge such interdependency. This country's mantra is that people are responsible for their own fates. Freedom is too often cast as being free to choose what's best for our own families and succeed for ourselves (and not having to think about how that choice impacts others), leaving others to their own separate fates and poor "choices." The stories in this book make it clear that vision of American freedom is dangerous and selfish, that individualistic ways of thinking and acting must change. We need a society with a different ethos, where we acknowledge what is happening to other people and imagine our relationships to them differently. We need to understand and act on the bonds of mutuality and reciprocity that connect us. As the group made clear we can't have a society where some people are sacrificed for the good of others and their suffering is kept out of sight. None of us are free until all of us are free. We need to acknowledge that the tales society tells—that the pandemic is over, that we celebrate and support essential workers, that the pandemic didn't discriminate—make it easier to avoid the profound asymmetries the pandemic exposed.

Our authors also insisted on the necessity of grieving, seeing grief as something that doesn't have a definitive end date. There is just so much loss and trauma to grapple with and mourn. You don't just get over such losses, our authors asserted; they stay with you and change you and the people and places around you. As of this writing, more than 1.1 million people in the United States have died; almost one sixth of the world's COVID deaths have taken place in this country. Lives have been lost, homes and apartments have been lost, as have good health, neighbors, and other forms of security. And our public conversation about COVID makes almost no space for grief and its reckonings. We are expected to muster forth, to forge ahead without looking back or taking stock of what and who has been lost.

This book, these writers insisted, is not a conclusion to the pandemic. It cannot be a conclusion. Despite the vaccines and boosters, the ending of the "national emergency" and mask mandates, despite the insistence that we can return to the way things were, we cannot. The pandemic lingers—both in the illness and death it continues to generate, and in the ripples of grief and aftereffects of hardship, struggle, fear, and heartbreak that reverberate, perhaps forever. We need to slow down, to acknowledge and process who has been hurt and who died, to reflect on what remains and what redress is needed and then engage in reparative action.

Part of the legacy of the pandemic for many of our writers is the mutual aid and grass-roots care and organizing that have taken place, providing food, shelter, medicine, and succor to people whom the state didn't do enough to protect. The networks forged and expanded during the pandemic showed the power of communities to protect their members, to help the most vulnerable. We are proud and inspired by the ways our communities acted when the state failed, they explained, feeling closer to neighbors as a result of these acts of solidarity and care.

But—and here the conversation took another turn—we can't just be talking about mutual aid and neighbors helping neighbors; we need structural change. One writer exclaimed: you can't mutual aid your way out of poverty and racism and a failing health care system. Our communities stepped up because the state failed and we didn't want our neighbors to starve or die. The pandemic showed the ways our communities came through when the state and corporations didn't, and that's always how it's been. But let's be clear: mutual aid is not the ultimate solution. The pandemic forced us to see the extremes of our society, the ways that our political system and economy are organized to make some people vulnerable and others much safer. All disparities were brought forth in the pandemic—from health to jobs, from benefits to housing to the environmental conditions we live in. As much as families can be sites of love and support, our social safety net cannot be the family alone. Our sustenance cannot be just our family's responsibility. Everyone we know worked hard, our writers underscored, and we deserve more than depending on the twenty dollars out of our neighbor's pocket, or a meal prepared by people who themselves are struggling to get by. The government has to do its part; we need an economy that is not organized to exploit the already vulnerable and enrich the already wealthy. It is not our responsibility alone to make sure we have decent lives.

We've known that the harmful policies and systems that create and exacerbate inequalities—racial capitalism foremost among them—have been around a long time and were created intentionally. It's not an accident, the authors asserted, that the perspectives we bring weren't heard. It's not an accident that poor and working people and immigrants were sacrificed for the well-being and profits of others. It's not an accident that many Americans wanted to make choices to have and do what they desired without having to think about the other people affected by those choices (and often get mad when they're pressed to do so). The pandemic exposed the cruel inequalities and mythologies that are baked into our society; it enabled—or forced—us to see the brutal human costs of the way we have set things up. We've seen how hard survival is: millions of people going into medical debt, people losing their homes, losing their jobs or deciding to quit to protect themselves and their loved ones, choosing between income and health, going hungry or losing their housing. The undocumented and BIPOC suffered more. All the while, the 1% made massive profits.

And while the pandemic brought inequality to the fore in public conversations for a time, many people have now chosen to look away; following the state's directives, the media have largely moved on. But that's not good enough, our writers argued. A public reckoning about what it would take to redress these drastic injustices is desperately needed—and then action. What it comes down to, these writers said, is living wages, actual hazard pay and paid sick leave, affordable housing and education for everyone, especially the people who faced (and continued to face) the hazards to put food on our tables, to protect and provide for our society's more well-off citizens. We know what it will take, we've been saying it, but people don't want to listen.

These ideas may seem overly idealistic, pie in the sky, but the pandemic also gave us a glimpse of what *is* possible and what *could* be done. Governments spent billions on new programs. They sent checks to citizens to provide some measure of relief for lost income (it was wholly inadequate, to be sure, but still invaluable; in some other countries, governments sent much more to their citizens). They put a halt on evictions, opened free testing and vaccine clinics, increased SNAP (Supplemental Nutrition Assistance Program), and expanded other food distribution programs. They sent testing kits to everyone through the mail (even when they had first mocked the idea). They did things we'd never seen; they showed us it *was* possible for local, state, and federal officials to act speedily to provide for people's needs.

Part of the stampede to return to normal is to make us forget that it is possible to do things differently. What would this country look like if we expanded and institutionalized these gestures of public support for collective well-being? Pandemic relief programs from food assistance to eviction moratoriums to paying rent for people who cannot afford it need to be made permanent. Funding for community-based organizations that are doing the work the city didn't also needs to be radically increased. We need much better regulations of job safety and *living* wages and jobs for everyone, our authors insisted. We need to protect not only renters but also prevent foreclosures—some homeowners need help paying the mortgage, too, and many homes in our neighborhoods have many generations living in them. Solve one issue, and you solve others, the student authors noted. If you solve food insecurity, you begin to solve public health; if you solve the housing affordability crisis, you start to solve public safety. The issues are inextricably linked together.

Many people today are still reeling from the hardships and heartbreak of the pandemic. They're taking grueling jobs at low wages to afford food on their table. People should not have to struggle to stay healthy, pay rent, and feed themselves and their families. Yet millions of Americans do, and the toll that takes goes largely unacknowledged. You should not have to go into debt to have housing, health, and education. Our authors agreed: we need universal health care, housing, education!

We need public access to mental health care as well as full medical health care because most of us can't afford therapy and mental health is overlooked. You're just supposed to tough it out, these writers explained—or when you do seek help, the therapists are white and make assumptions about your family and community. Yet mental health struggles are not just a personal matter but connected to the way our society is structured. We need regular mental health check-ins and some form of free therapy for all public workers. We need community centers that help support mental health literacy. And we need housing, food, jobs, health care—and a society working to eradicate racism, homophobia, transphobia, anti-immigrant bias and misogyny—because these are crucial linchpins to our mental health.

But, another student-scholar interjected, we can't simply improve and expand existing policies because they often leave undocumented people out. We need to change our immigration system. Currently, undocumented people are not eligible for many programs and benefits. One author asked: How can we imagine safety for people who are in occupied territories? Other contributors asserted that people must be enfranchised to determine what is best for them where they live. People need access to health care, housing, and jobs regardless of citizenship status.

Others in the conversation noted that new policies in and of themselves are not enough. We also need a new policy process, in which directly affected communities—those who have suffered the most under our current arrangements—make, test, and evaluate policies. The realities we documented need to be front and center in terms of building solutions. We cannot leave policy to the politicians but need truly participatory democracy, not the top-down policymaking that passes for democracy in our current system. We must work to collectively ensure that everyone has a say in crafting the policies that shape their lives through community-controlled institutions and participatory democracy. This book is one effort to amplify voices that are regularly ignored in our society and insist they be centered in public policy. But a book can only do so much; real change through collective action is required.

We are not concluding. This is a call to see, to bear witness, and then to act. The ideas presented here are the fruit of years of thought and experience and one afternoon's conversation together with these writers. But they are not a policy brief. Rather, this is an invitation and insistence to you, our readers, to consider these uncomfortable truths and then find collective ways of making critical change and justice happen. There is so much desire in the United States to go back to normal and call the pandemic over. Yet the way things are now is nowhere near good enough. Perhaps the idea of the normal—that there is a *norm*, that one size fits all—is part of the problem. We need a system, a society, that can account for the full, rich diversity and variety of our lives and redress and repair the historical inequalities—of race, gender, class, immigration, nationality, disability, and more—that have made the pandemic and the present so painful and so unfair.

When we are truly seen, the student contributors in this book collectively assert, we cannot continue this way. Where we go from here is up to all of us.

NOTES

Introduction

1. Dave Lucas, "Gov. Delivers Labor Day Address to New Yorkers," WAMC Northeast Public Radio, September 7, 2020, https://www.wamc.org/new-york-news/2020-09-07/gov-delivers-labor-day-address-to-new-yorkers.

2. University of Pennsylvania Press style typically uses italics as a way to mark people speaking and also for sentences or phrases in a foreign language. They did not require translating any of the Spanish—which we very much appreciated. Any time translation is provided in a chapter, it is because the author wanted to provide it. Still, the use of italics has the potential to seem otherizing, which our authors noted and so the press allowed us to remove the italics.

3. See: "COVID-19 and the Social Sciences," Social Science Research Council, https://COVID19research.ssrc.org/.

4. The pieces from the summer 2020 cohort are archived at SSRC here: https://inequality-initiative.ssrc.org/autoethnographies-of-a-pandemic-from-brooklyns-epicenter/.

5. This second cohort was funded by Brooklyn College and the third cohort was funded by the Andrew W. Mellon Foundation.

6. In January 2021, *Popular Science* and *American Prospect* declared Los Angeles the "new epicenter of COVID-19." Sara Chodosh, "5 Graphs That Show How Bad COVID-19 is in LA County," *Popular Science*, January 25, 2021; Harold Myerson, "Why COVID-19 Has Run Amok in Los Angeles," *American Prospect*, January 25, 2021.

7. Full report here: "During the COVID-19 Pandemic, People of Color Were More Likely to Die at Younger Ages," KFF News release, April 24, 2023, https://www.kff.org/coronavirus-COVID-19/press-release/during-the-COVID-19-pandemic-people-of-color-were-more-likely-to-die-at-younger-ages/.

8. See "CUNY's Contribution to the Economy," New York City Comptroller, https://comptroller.nyc.gov/reports/cunys-contribution-to-the-economy/#:~:text=Over%2080%20percent%20of%20incoming,households%20with%20incomes%20below%20%2430%2C000 and "2016 Student Experience Survey," Office of Institutional Research and Assessment, https://www.cuny.edu/wp-content/uploads/sites/4/page-assets/about/administration/offices/oira/institutional/surveys/2016_SES_Highlights_Updated_web_ready.pdf.

9. Ben Chapman, "Thousands of CUNY Students Experience Homelessness and Food Insecurity, Report Says," *New York Daily News*, March 27, 2019.

10. Heidi E. Jones et al., "The Impact of the COVID-19 Pandemic on College Students' Health and Financial Stability in New York City: Findings from a Population-Based Sample of City University of New York (CUNY) Students," *Journal of Urban Health* 98 (2021): 187–96, https://link.springer.com/article/10.1007/s11524-020-00506-x.

11. Data at: "Economic Diversity and Student Outcomes at California State University, Los Angeles," *New York Times*, https://www.nytimes.com/interactive/projects/college-mobility/california-state-university-los-angeles.

12. Janice Carr, "CSULB Associate Professor Inspires $15 Million CSU Grant to Combat Student Food, Housing Insecurity," *LB News*, November 29, 2021, https://www.csulb.edu/news/article/csulb-associate-professor-inspires-15-million-csu-grant-to-combat-student-food-housing.

13. https://www.csac.ca.gov/sites/main/files/file-attachments/fall_2020_covid19_student_survey_results_presentation.pdf.

14. Debbie Truong, "Cal State Details Potential Tuition Increases amid Massive Funding Gap," *Los Angeles Times*, June 6, 2023.

15. Barbara Jacoby, "What about the Other 85%?" *Inside Higher Ed*, July 23, 2020.

16. As of the fall 2022 semester, this requirement has, at last, been revised so that part-time students are now eligible for state tuition assistance.

17. Alan Aja, Joseph Entin, and Jeanne Theoharis, "The True Crime in Higher Education: How We've Abandoned Public Universities like CUNY," *New York Daily News*, April 2, 2019.

18. Jesse McKinley, "New York City Region Is Now an Epicenter of the Coronavirus Pandemic," *New York Times*, March 22, 2020.

19. "New York City Coronavirus Map and Case Count," *New York Times*, May 9, 2020.

20. Naomi Singer, "Disproportionate Impact of COVID-19 on Lower-Income, Minority Populations," *Ohio Journal of Public Health* 3, no. 3 (December 2020): 3–5.

21. "Inequities in Experiences of the COVID-19 Pandemic, New York City," EPI Data Brief, NYC Health, https://www1.nyc.gov/assets/doh/downloads/pdf/epi/data-brief123.pdf.

22. "Excluded in the Epicenter: Impact of the COVID Crisis on Working-Class Immigrant, Black, and Brown New Yorkers," Make the Road New York, May 2020, https://maketheroadny.org/wp-content/uploads/2020/05/MRNY_SurveyReport_small.pdf.

23. Diana-Lyn Baptiste et al., "COVID-19: Shedding Light on Racial and Health Inequities in the USA," *Journal of Clinical Nursing*, June 14, 2020, https://www.ncbi.nlm.nih.gov/pmc/articles/PMC7300762/#jocn15351-bib-0019.

24. Ibid.

25. Irene Lew, "Race and the Economic Fallout from COVID-19 in New York City," Community Service Society Report, June 30, 2020, https://www.cssny.org/news/entry/race-and-the-economic-fallout-from-COVID-19-in-new-york-city.

26. Emily Benfer et al., "Eviction, Health Inequity, and the Spread of COVID-19: Housing Policy as a Primary Pandemic Mitigation Strategy," *Journal of Urban Health* 98, no. 1 (February 2021): 1–12, https://www.ncbi.nlm.nih.gov/pmc/articles/PMC7790520/#CR10.

27. William Guillaume Koible and Insiah Figueroa, "Fighting More Than COVID-19: Unmasking the State of Hunger in NYC During a Pandemic," foodbanknyc.org, June 2020.

28. Rachel Tillman, "Report: Hate crimes rose 44% last year in study of major cities," February 15, 2022, *Spectrum News, NY1*, https://www.ny1.com/nyc/all-boroughs/news/2022/02/14/hate-crime-increase-2021-asian-american-.

29. "Police Killed 164 Black People in the First 8 Months of 2020. These Are Their Names," CBS News, September 10, 2020, https://www.cbsnews.com/pictures/black-people-killed-by-police-in-the-u-s-in-2020/.

30. As of July 2022, New York City, with a population of just over 8 million residents, has reported 5.7 million cases and over 69,000 deaths. The daily average on July 18, 2022—7,712 cases per day—was roughly the same daily infection rate as April 20, 2020, when 7,662 cases were reported. The death rate, however, had dropped substantially from April 2020 to July 2022.

31. As a 2022 Oxfam report notes: "The world's ten richest men more than doubled their fortunes from $700 billion to $1.5 trillion—at a rate of $15,000 per second or $1.3 billion a day—during the first two years of a pandemic that has seen the incomes of 99 percent of humanity fall and over 160 million more people forced into poverty."

32. Laura Nahmias, "New York City's New Mayor Tells the City It's Time to Stop Wallowing in COVID," *Bloomberg News*, January 11, 2022.

33. New York data can be found here: https://coronavirus.health.ny.gov/covid-19-wastewater-surveillance-weekly-summary-report.

34. "Turning a Second Home into a Primary Home," *New York Times*, July 24, 2020.

35. The United States had the highest COVID death rate among highly industrialized countries; one study "estimated that a single-payer universal healthcare system would have saved 212,000 lives in 2020 alone." "UN Could Have Saved 338,000 Lives from COVID with Universal Health Care," *Guardian*, June 16, 2022.

36. Ruth Wilson Gilmore defines racism as "the state-sanctioned and/or extra-legal production and exploitation of group-differentiated vulnerability to premature death," Gilmore, *Golden Gulag: Prisons, Surplus, Crisis, and Opposition in Globalizing California* (Berkeley: University of California Press, 2006), 28.

37. Paul Fronstin and Steven A. Woodbury, "How Many Americans Have Lost Jobs with Employer Health Coverage During the Pandemic?," The Commonwealth Fund Issue Brief, October 7, 2020, https://www.commonwealthfund.org/publications/issue-briefs/2020/oct/how-many-lost-jobs-employer-coverage-pandemic.

38. Chuck Collins, "US Billionaires Got 62 Percent Richer During Pandemic. They're Now Up $1.8 Trillion," Institute for Policy Studies, August 24, 2021, https://ips

-dc.org/u-s-billionaires-62-percent-richer-during-pandemic/. This book makes a differ-ent contribution to the growing number of books about the pandemic, such as Thomas J. Sugrue and Cailtin Zaloom, eds., *The Long Year: A 2020 Reader* (New York: Columbia University Press, 2022), Rhae Lynn Barnes, Keri Leigh Merritt, and Yohuru Williams, eds., *After Life: A Collective History of Loss and Redemption in Pandemic America* (New York: Haymarket, 2022), and Dao X. Tran, ed., *Unheard Voices of the Pandemic: Narra-tive from the First Year of COVID-19* (New York: Haymarket, 2021) by foregrounding student researchers from directly affected communities who provide a granular, tex-tured analysis of those inequalities from the ground up.

39. Audre Lorde, "Learning from the 1960s," address at Harvard University: https://www.blackpast.org/african-american-history/1982-audre-lorde-learning-60s/.

Chapter 1

1. Rachel Garfield, "Double Jeopardy: Low Wage Workers at Risk for Health and Financial Implications of COVID-19," Kaiser Family Foundation, April 29, 2020: https://www.kff.org/coronavirus-COVID-19/issue-brief/double-jeopardy-low-wage-workers-at-risk-for-health-and-financial-implications-of-COVID-19/.

2. Alexina Cather and Heidi Andrianos, "Fast Food Wage War and Strikes in New York City: A Timeline," NYC Food Policy Center (Hunter College), September 26, 2018.

3. Living wage calculator here: https://livingwage.mit.edu/.

4. "As Coronavirus Spreads, Which US Workers Have Paid Sick Leave—and Which Don't?," Pew Research Center, March 12, 2020, https://www.pewresearch.org/fact-tank/2020/03/12/as-coronavirus-spreads-which-u-s-workers-have-paid-sick-leave-and-which-dont/.

5. "McDonald's Employees are Working through the COVID-19 Pandemic. So Why Don't They Have Access to Paid Sick and Family Leave?," ACLU Report, May 1, 2020, https://www.aclu.org/news/racial-justice/mcdonalds-employees-are-working-through-the-COVID-19-pandemic-so-why-dont-they-have-access-to-paid-sick-and-family-leave/.

6. Garfield, "Double Jeopardy: Low Wage Workers at Risk."

7. "Silenced About COVID-19 in the Workplace," National Employment Law Proj-ect, June 2020, https://s27147.pcdn.co/wp-content/uploads/Silenced-About-COVID-19-Workplace-Fear-Retaliation-June-2020.pdf.

8. "How State and Local Governments Can Support Safe Workplaces and Protect Public Health During the Coronavirus Crisis," Center for the American Prospect Action Fund, May 13, 2020, https://www.americanprogressaction.org/issues/economy/news/2020/05/13/177671/state-local-governments-can-support-safe-workplaces-protect-public-health-coronavirus-crisis/.

9. Carlie Porterfield, "No-Mask Attacks: Nationwide, Employees Face Violence for Enforcing Mask Mandates," *Forbes*, August 15, 2020.

10. "Making Ends Meet in the Margins: Female-Dominated, Low-Wage Sectors," *New America*, September 26, 2018.

Chapter 2

1. Jerilyn Jordan, "Dildos Are Non-Essential, Amazon Worker Says, as Romulus Facility Protests Conditions amid Coronavirus Crisis," *Detroit Metro Times*, April 6, 2020.

2. Ken Schachter, "Amazon: New Facility Will 'Primarily Serve' LI," *Newsday*, April 27, 2016.

3. Shelley E. Kohan, "Amazon's Net Profit Soars 84% with Sales Hitting $386 Billion," *Forbes*, December 10, 2021.

4. Jay Greene, "Amazon's Big Holiday Shopping Advantage: An In-House Shipping Network Swollen by Pandemic-Fueled Growth," *Washington Post*, November 28, 2020.

5. Lauren Kaori Gurley, "Amazon 'Delivery Partners' Hit Amazon with $15 Million Lawsuit," *VICE*, October 27, 2021.

6. Irina Ivanova, "Amazon Fires Worker Who Organized Staten Island Warehouse Walkout," *CBS News*, March 30, 2020.

7. Julia Carrie Wong, "Amazon Execs Labeled Fired Worker 'Not Smart or Articulate' in Leaked PR Notes," *Guardian*, April 2, 2020.

8. Andrea Hsu, "In a Stunning Victory, Amazon Workers on Staten Island Vote for a Union," *NPR*, April 1, 2022.

9. Michael Sheetz, "Jeff Bezos Says Sales of Blue Origin Space Tourist Flights Are 'Approaching $100 Million' Already," *CNBC*, July 20, 2021.

10. William Harwood, "Jeff Bezos and Blue Origin Complete Successful Spaceflight," *CBS News*, July 21, 2021.

11. Chase Peterson-Withorn, "Led by Elon Musk's Crazy Gains, American Billionaires Have Added Nearly $2 Trillion to Their Fortunes during the Pandemic," *Forbes*, November 8, 2021.

12. Jason Del Rey, "Amazon's Worker Union Just Lost in New York City. Where Does It Go from Here?," *Vox*, May 2, 2022.

Chapter 3

1. "COVID-19 Deaths Analyzed by Race and Ethnicity," APM Research Lab, https://www.apmresearchlab.org/COVID/deaths-by-race.

2. Elisa Gould and Valerie Wilson, "Black Workers Face Two of the Most Lethal Preexisting Conditions for Coronavirus—Racism and Economic Inequality," Economic Policy Institute, June 1, 2020, https://www.epi.org/publication/black-workers-COVID/.

3. Ibid.

4. Latoya Hill (@hill_latoya) and Samantha Artiga (@SArtiga2), Twitter, February 22, 2022; "COVID-19 Cases and Deaths by Race/Ethnicity: Current Data and Changes Over Time, KFF issue brief, https://www.kff.org/coronavirus-COVID-19/issue-brief/COVID-19-cases-and-deaths-by-race-ethnicity-current-data-and-changes-over-time/.

5. "New York City's Frontline Workers," March 26, 2020, New York City Comptroller, https://comptroller.nyc.gov/reports/new-york-citys-frontline-workers/.

6. Gould and Wilson, "Black Workers."

Chapter 4

1. Karen Hacker et al., "Barriers to Health Care for Undocumented Immigrants: A Literature Review," *Risk Management and Healthcare Policy 8* (October 30, 2015): 175–83.

2. Rachel Holliday Smith, "Chicken, Plantains and Café Bustelo: Uplift NYC Pivots to Help Uptown Families," *The City*, May 11, 2020, https://www.thecity.nyc/corona virus/2020/5/11/21257152/chicken-plantains-and-cafe-bustelo-uplift-nyc-pivots-to -help-uptown-families.

3. "Undocumented Essential Workers: 5 Things to Know," Fwd.us, February 8, 2021, https://www.fwd.us/news/undocumented-essential-workers-5-things-to-know/.

4. James Parrott and Lina Moe, "The New Strain of Inequality: The Economic Impact of COVID-19 in New York City," Center for New York City Affairs report, April 15, 2020.

5. "Married to an Undocumented Immigrant? You May Not Get a Stimulus Check," *New York Times*, April 28, 2020.

6. Daniel Gross, "The Transformation of Hart Island: The Coronavirus Is Permanently Changing the Role of New York City's Public Burial Ground," *New Yorker*, April 10, 2020.

7. "City Cemetery Hart Island (Potter's Field)." Correction Department, City of New York, http://www.correctionhistory.org/html/chronicl/nycdoc/html/hart.html.

8. D. E. Slotnik, "Up to a Tenth of New York City's Coronavirus Dead May Be Buried in a Potter's Field," *New York Times*, March 25, 2021.

9. W. J. Hennigan. "Inside New York City's Mass Graveyard on Hart Island." *Time*, November 19, 2020.

Chapter 5

1. See for instance, Maria Pérez y González and Virginia Sánchez-Korrol, eds., *Puerto Rican Studies: The First Fifty Years* (New York: Centro Press, 2021).

2. A classic piece by Pedro Caban, "Moving from the Margins to Where? Three Decades of Latino/a Studies," *Journal of Latino Studies* 1 (2003), maps a pre-millennium trajectory of Latinx Studies that is still quite relevant two decades later. He highlights three types of existing, interacting models—the enclave (tolerated by the institution but heavily underfunded), the transgressive (possessing intellectual authority and well funded) and absorption (merged with other area studies with minimal resources/curricular offerings). I would argue our department exists within the "enclave Latino Studies" model, where a department carries out its work while chronically fiscally marginalized and understaffed.

3. For further context, CUNY runs on an immoral fiduciary model where student tuition dollars are used to make up for inadequate state- to city-level funding, thus college administrations see students as "revenue." A policy-level counter to this model, a *New Deal for CUNY*, is currently on the table in the New York state legislature, which would eliminate tuition and fees for in-state students and replace tuition-revenue with federal, state, and local monies.

4. One of the student speakers at this rally, Daniel Vázquez Sanabria, and a faculty speaker, Lawrence Johnson, are contributors to this book. Both were part of a campus-wide Anti-Racist Coalition that Rhea Rahman also writes about that was created in the wake of the George Floyd and Breonna Taylor protests to demand a transformative over-haul of the college's spending and disciplinary priorities.

5. Ken Klippenstein and Jon Schwarz, "Bank of America Memo, Revealed: 'We Hope' Conditions for American Workers Will Get Worse," *Intercept*, July 29, 2022, https://theintercept.com/2022/07/29/bank-of-america-worker-conditions-worse/.

6. A large part of how banks profited is through the designed structure and rules of pandemic stimulus measures from the federal government (central bank). Suppos-edly designed to "bail out" everyday people, instead capital flowed upward to large cor-porations and bond holders. See for example: John Cassidy, "Wall Street's Pandemic Bonanza," *New Yorker*, January 18, 2022; Jesse Eisinger, "The Bailout Is Working—for the Rich," *ProPublica*, May 10, 2020.

7. In fact, the same internal memo admits the bank's anxiety over increasing worker power, stating that a "record tight labor market" and higher wages is going "to be hard to reverse." See Klippenstein and Schwarz, 1.

8. Sometimes the predominant view spills into romanticized narratives of tony resi-dential campuses where students live and study without financial worry (narratives that erase working-class students in those very elite spaces, not to mention the amount of student debt students of color often accrue to attend those elite schools). For more on the latter, see Santul Nerkar, "Canceling Student Debt Could Help Close the Wealth Gap," *FiveThirtyEight*, May 31, 2022.

9. Laura W. Perna and Taylor K. Odle, "Recognizing the Reality of Working College Students," *Academe*, Vol. 106, No. 1 (Winter 2020), "The Social Mission of Higher Edu-cation." The report, published amid the first year of the pandemic, cited US Department of Education employment data from 2017. It demonstrated that 43% of full-time under-graduate students and an astonishing 81% of part-time undergraduates were employed while attending school.

10. From what I have seen, administrative decision-makers readily acknowledge that CUNY students rely on work to afford the aforementioned rising costs of education and that work is often an inflexible barrier to registering for the right courses needed to graduate and to overall academic performance. Despite this, fiscal justice-based policy is rarely the response.

11. This term is also inspired by the work of the late, great Juan Flores, whose book *Diaspora Strikes Back: Caribeño Tales of Learning and Turning* (New York: Routledge, 2009), remains a quintessential analysis in the Puerto Rican and Latinx Studies literature.

12. Here I refer to the growing "credentialing" literature—specifically the reality that people of color, in order to compensate for the labor market discrimination they encounter, "over-credential" (invest in even more education, training) to experience the same returns as the dominant, non-racially discriminated group (whites). See for example Tressie McMillan-Cottom, *Lower Ed: The Troubling Rise of For-Profit Colleges*

in the New Economy (New York: The New Press, 2018). Also see Janelle Jones and John Schmitt, "A College Degree Is No Guarantee," Center for Economic and Policy Research, 2014, https://cepr.net/report/a-college-degree-is-no-guarantee/. On student debt, see for example Louise Seamster and Alan Aja, "A Regressive Student Loan System Results in Costly Disparities," Brookings, *Still We Rise Blog*, January 24, 2022.

13. For an alternative take-down of "human capital theory," see the emerging field of "stratification economics," which emphasizes resource-level disparities, intergenerational transmissions (wealth inequality), group positionality, and discrimination as factors explaining social and economic disparities. See Kate Bahn and Carmen Sanchez Cumming, "Stratification Economics: What It Is and How It Advances Our Understanding of Inequality," Washington Center for Equitable Growth, February 28, 2022. Also further note, in Los Angeles county specifically, a recent report by the UCLA Labor Center underscored that the overwhelming majority of young workers of color work to support their families, pay for their education, and purchase basic living needs. The report also noted that they experience higher levels of unemployment and low wages even in the possession of college degrees. See Reyna Orellana, Jeylee Quiroz, and Monica Macias, "Young Workers in California: A Snapshot," UCLA Labor Center, March 2020, https://www.labor.ucla.edu/publication/young-workers-in-california-a-snapshot -young-workers-animated-for-change-workshop-and-classroom-guide/.

14. Roberto Suro and Hanna Findling, "New York's Essential Workers: Overlooked, Underpaid, and Indispensable," Fiscal Policy Institute, April 2020, http://fiscalpolicy.org /wp-content/uploads/2020/04/Essential-Workers-Brief-Final-1.pdf.

15. See Celine McNicholas and Margaret Poydock, "Who Are Essential Workers? A Comprehensive Look at Their Wages, Demographics, and Unionization Rates," Economic Policy Institute, May 19, 2020, https://www.epi.org/blog/who-are-essential-work-ers-a-comprehensive-look-at-their-wages-demographics-and-unionization-rates/.

16. Prior to the pandemic, an emergent literature on "precarious work" shed light on its wide effects on the physical and mental health of workers, with disproportionate impact on workers of color. Relatedly here, it is important to point out that historically Black unemployment has been persistently twice the rate of whites, a material reality that has been lost amid the "pre-pandemic" analyses. For a good summary of this reality, see Pavlina Tcherneva, "Controlling the Viral Spread of Unemployment via a Job Guarantee," *American Prospect,* June 26, 2020.

17. For instance, Chris Famighetti and Darrick Hamilton highlight the ways the overall reduction of wealth since the Great Recession was not experienced similarly across racial and ethnic groups. Related to education, whereas they point out that "a college degree is often framed as a reliable stepping stone on the path to economic security," they found that Black college graduates experienced more barriers to the housing market relative to other groups. See Chris Famighetti and Darrick Hamilton, "The Great Recession, Race and Home Ownership," Economic Policy Institute, May 15, 2019, https://www.epi.org/blog/the-great-recession-education-race-and-homeownership/.

18. See for example Jeanne Smialek, "The Fed Eyes a Hot Labor Market as Unemployment Nears Pre-pandemic Levels," *New York Times*, April 1, 2022.

19. See for instance Ira Katznelson, *When Affirmative Action was White* (New York: W.W. Norton, 2006) for an analysis of how the New Deal and subsequent asset-building policies (the very same program that funded the building of three CUNY campuses) were implemented in a racially discriminatory manner.

20. Tania further aims her critique at the brutality of work in America, stating powerfully: "My father has worked constantly since he migrated from Haiti and has only called in sick once for emergency appendix surgery. That was only after he completed his shift and drove himself to the hospital, where he was forced to take a couple of days off to recover. If that doesn't illustrate the lack of economic security and compassion in America for the working people, I don't know what does."

21. McNicholas and Poydoc, "Who Are Essential Workers?"

22. The term "everyday revolutions" has been used by several writers, but I'm referring here to the way sociologist-lawyer-activist Marina Sitrin applied it to her observations in Argentina after the global financial crisis as new forms of social organizations began to formulate. See Marina Sitrin, *Everyday Revolutions: Horizontalism and Autonomy in Argentina* (New York: Zed books, 2012).

Chapter 6

1. Julia Ries. "COVID-19 Has Serious Effects on People with Severe Mental Illness," *Healthline*, April 7, 2020.

2. American Psychiatric Association, "Mental Health Disparities: African Americans," https://www.psychiatry.org/File%20Library/Psychiatrists/Cultural-Competency/Mental-Health-Disparities/Mental-Health-Facts-for-African-Americans.pdf

3. Darcel Rockett, "Black Mental Health Patients Hit Hard by COVID-19, Social Injustice: 'We Were Already at a Breaking Point,'" *Chicago Tribune*, July 15, 2020.

4. "The COVID Racial Data Tracker," The COVID Tracking Project, https://COVIDtracking.com/race.

Chapter 7

1. "Public Charge," US Citizenship and Immigration Services, https://www.uscis.gov/public-charge.

2. Erika Lee, *America for Americans: A History of Xenophobia in the United States* (Basic Books, 2019), 49.

3. Kathryn Olivarius, "The Dangerous History of Immunoprivilege," *New York Times*, April 12, 2020.

4. Ibid.

5. US Immigration and Customs Enforcement, *Fiscal Year 2020 Enforcement and Removal Operations Report*, December 23, 2020, 19, https://www.ice.gov/doclib/news/library/reports/annual-report/iceReportFY2020.pdf.

6. Miles Parks et al., "Trump Signs Order to End Family Separations," *NPR*, June 20, 2018.

7. "US: New Report Shines Spotlight on Abuses and Growth in Immigrant Detention Under Trump," April 30, 2020, Human Rights Watch, https://www.hrw.org/news/2020/04/30/us-new-report-shines-spotlight-abuses-and-growth-immigrant-detention-under-trump.

8. Dara Lind and Lomi Kriel, "ICE Is Making Sure Migrant Kids Don't Have COVID-19—Then Expelling Them to 'Prevent the Spread' of COVID-19," *ProPublica*, August 10, 2020, https://www.propublica.org/article/ice-is-making-sure-migrant-kids-dont-have-covid-19-then-expelling-them-to-prevent-the-spread-of-covid-19.

9. "The US Detained Hundreds of Migrant Children in Hotels as the Pandemic Flared," *CNN*, September 3, 2020.

10. Ibid.

11. Lind and Kriel, "ICE Is Making Sure Migrant Kids Don't Have COVID-19."

12. Jacob Soboroff, *Separated: Inside an American Tragedy* (New York: Custom House, 2020), 70.

13. Andrew Glass, "Bush Creates Homeland Security Department," *Politico*, November 26, 2002, https://www.politico.com/story/2018/11/26/this-day-in-politics-november-26-1012269.

14. Alejandra Marchevsky and Beth Baker, "Why Has President Obama Deported More Immigrants Than Any in History," *Nation*, March 31, 2014.

15. "Remarks by the President on Comprehensive Immigration Reform," The White House, retrieved July 20, 2021, https://obamawhitehouse.archives.gov/realitycheck/node/14130.

16. "DHS Proposes Fair and Humane Public Charge Rule," February 17, 2022, https://www.uscis.gov/newsroom/news-releases/dhs-proposes-fair-and-humane-public-charge-rule; and "Public Charge Ground of Inadmissibility," posted by the US Citizenship and Immigration Services on February 24, 2022, https://www.regulations.gov/document/USCIS-2021-0013-0198.

Chapter 8

1. US Immigration and Customs Enforcement, "FY20 ICE Detention Statistics," https://www.ice.gov/detain/detention-management.

2. "COVID-19 Escalating in ICE Detention Centers as States Hit Highest Daily Records—and ICE Deportation Flights into Northern Triangle Continue," International Rescue Committee, August 3, 2020, https://www.rescue.org/press-release/COVID-19-escalating-ice-detention-centers-states-hit-highest-daily-records-and-ice.

3. John Washington, "ICE Mismanagement Created Coronavirus 'Hotbeds of Infection' in and around Detention Centers," *Intercept*, December 9, 2020; and "COVID-19 Escalating in ICE Detention Centers as States Hit Highest Daily Records."

4. Dan Glaun, "How ICE Data Undercounts COVID-19 Victim," *Frontline*, August 11, 2020, https://www.pbs.org/wgbh/frontline/article/how-ice-data-undercounts-COVID-19-victims/.

5. Butler County Sheriff's Office, "First Confirmed COVID-19 Case in Butler County Jail" (press release), April 13, 2020, http://www.butlersheriff.org/2020/04/13/first-confirmed-COVID-19-case-in-butler-county-jail/.

6. "COVID-19 Escalating in ICE Detention Centers."

7. John Washington, "ICE Mismanagement Created Coronavirus 'Hotbeds of Infection' in and around Detention Centers," *Intercept*, December 9, 2020, https://theintercept.com/2020/12/09/ice-covid-detention-centers/.

8. Glaun, "How ICE Data Undercounts COVID-19 Victim."

9. Washington, "ICE Mismanagement Created Coronavirus 'Hotbeds.'"

10. Ibid.

Chapter 9

1. Katie Rogers et al., "Trump Defends Using 'Chinese Virus' Label, Ignoring Growing Criticism," *New York Times*, March 18, 2020.

2. Claire Ewing-Nelson, "All of the Jobs Lost in December Were Women's Jobs," National Women's Law Center, January 2021, https://nwlc.org/wp-content/uploads/2021/01/December-Jobs-Day.pdf; Rakesh Kochhar and Anthony Cilluffo, "Income Inequality in the US Is Rising Most Rapidly Among Asians," Pew Research Center's Social and Demographic Trends Project, July 12, 2018, https://www.pewresearch.org/social-trends/2018/07/12/income-inequality-in-the-u-s-is-rising-most-rapidly-among-asians/.

3. "The Impact of COVID-19 on Asian American Employment in NYC," Asian American Foundation, https://aafCOVID19resourcecenter.org/unemployment-report/.

4. Kara Chin, Amelia Kosciulek, and Mark Abadi, "2 Organizations Are Working to Revive NYC's Chinatown as It Reels from the Pandemic and Racial Stigma," *Business Insider*, August 5, 2020.

5. Donald Mar and Paul Ong, *COVID-19's Employment Disruptions to Asian Americans*, UCLA Asian American Studies Center, July 20, 2020, http://www.aasc.ucla.edu/resources/policyreports/COVID19_Employment_CNK-AASC_072020.pdf.

6. "NYC LMI Storefront Loan," *NYC Business*; Tanay Warerkar, "Chinatown Businesses Frustrated over Exclusion from NYC COVID-19 Loan Program," *Eater NY*, January 5, 2021, https://ny.eater.com/2021/1/5/22213569/chinatown-loan-small-business-COVID-19-relief.

7. "State of New York Pandemic Small Business Recovery Grant Program," Empire State Development, accessed July 8, 2021, https://nysmallbusinessrecovery.com/.

8. Alyssa Paolicelli, "Mayor Seen in Video Turning Back on Chinatown Bakery Owner's Plea for Help," *Spectrum News NY1*, August 14, 2020.

9. "Announcing the LONGEVITY Fund: Welcome to Chinatown's Small Business Relief Fund," Welcome to Chinatown, July 17, 2020, https://www.welcometochinatown

.com/news/announcing-the-longevity-fund-welcome-to-chinatowns-small-business
-relief-fund.

10. Chin et al., "2 Organizations Are Working to Revive NYC's Chinatown."

11. Neil G. Ruiz, Juliana Menasce, and Christine Tamir, "Many Black, Asian Americans Say They Have Experienced Discrimination Amid Coronavirus," Pew Research Center's Social & Demographic Trends Project, July 1, 2020, https://www.pewresearch .org/social-trends/2020/07/01/many-black-and-asian-americans-say-they-have -experienced-discrimination-amid-the-COVID-19-outbreak/.

12. Neil G. Ruiz, Khadjiah Edwards, and Mark Hugo Lopez, "One-Third of Asian Americans Fear Threats, Physical Attacks and Most Say Violence against Them Is Rising," Pew Research Center, April 21, 2012, https://www.pewresearch.org/fact-tank/2021/04 /21/one-third-of-asian-americans-fear-threats-physical-attacks-and-most-say-violence -against-them-is-rising/.

13. Paolicelli, "Mayor Seen in Video Turning Back."

14. "Mayor de Blasio and Taskforce on Racial Inclusion & Equity Announce Expansion of NYC Care and Mental Health Services to Address Disparate Impact of COVID-19 on People of Color," Official Website of the City of New York, June 9, 2020, https://www1.nyc.gov/office-of-the-mayor/news/423-20/mayor-de-blasio-taskforce -racial-inclusion-equity-expansion-nyc-care-and.

15. Rong Xiaoqing, "First Lady Apologizes for Mwbe Language Excluding Asians." *City Limits*, September 2, 2020.

16. CeFaan Kim, "Exclusive Video: 52-Year-Old Asian Woman Violently Shoved Yesterday in Flushing, Queens," Twitter, February 17, 2021, https://twitter.com/CeFaan Kim/status/1362192082924896256.

17. Safewalx, https://safewalx.com.

18. Connie Hanzhang Jin, "6 Charts That Dismantle the Trope of Asian Americans as a Model Minority." NPR, May 25, 2021; William McGurn, "Opinion: The Woke 'Model Minority' Myth," *Wall Street Journal*, February 22, 2021.

19. Denise Lu, et al., "Faces of Power: 80% Are White, Even as US Becomes More Diverse." *New York Times*, September 10, 2020.

Chapter 10

1. Matthew Countryman, "2020 Uprisings, Unprecedented in Scope, Join a Long River of Struggle in America," *The Conversation*, June 7, 2020, https://theconversation .com/2020-uprisings-unprecedented-in-scope-join-a-long-river-of-struggle-in-america -139853.

2. Vincent Barone, "NYPD Officer Rams into Crowd of George Floyd Protesters in Brooklyn," *New York Post,* May 30, 2020.

3. Emma Specter, "Governor Cuomo Has Announced an 11 p.m. Curfew for New York City," *Vogue*, June 1, 2020.

4. Megan Burney, "UPDATED: Black Lives Matter Protest Schedule for June 6, 2020," *Bushwick Daily*, June 6, 2020.

5. Zackary Okun Dunivin et al., "Black Lives Matter Protests Shift Public Discourse," *Proceedings of the National Academy of Sciences* 119, no. 10 (March 8, 2022).

6. In *What Is Antiracism? And Why It Means Anticapitalism* (London: Verso, 2023), Arun Kundnani distinguishes between the radical antiracism that brought people to the streets in the uprising of 2020, versus a liberal antiracism adopted by universities, corporations, and government departments, in response. Whereas the former understood racism as structural and demanded the dismantling rather than reform of infrastructures of violence, the latter focused on micro-aggressions of individual biases. Kundnani explains the inadequacy of liberal antiracism: "Without an explanation of what the *structure* in structural racism is, these accounts cannot explain what sustains the unconscious biases they see as so damaging" (11).

7. Christen A. Smith, "Slow Death: Is the Trauma of Police Violence Killing Black Women?," *The Conversation*, July 11, 2016, https://theconversation.com/slow-death-is -the-trauma-of-police-violence-killing-black-women-62264.

8. Claire Colebrook, "Fast Violence, Revolutionary Violence: Black Lives Matter and the 2020 Pandemic," *Journal of Bioethical Inquiry* 17, no. 4 (2020): 495–99.

9. Ruth Wilson Gilmore and Beatrice Adler-Bolton, "Organized Abandonment w/ Ruth Wilson Gilmore," Death Panel Podcast, October 6, 2022, https://www.death panel.net/transcripts/organized-abandonment-with-ruth-wilson-gilmore.

10. Tom Kertscher, "No, Black Lives Matter Is Not a Terrorist Organization," Politi-Fact, July 20, 2020, https://www.politifact.com/factchecks/2020/jul/30/facebook-posts /black-lives-matter-not-terrorist-organization/.

11. As many of the authors in this volume also recognize, Gilmore's conception has gained traction as a particularly useful way to understand the state's response (and lack thereof) to the pandemic.

12. "Call for papers for the Canadian Association of Cultural Studies conference Organized Abandonment: Cultures of Crisis and Resistance at Simon Fraser University, May 15–16, 2020," https://www.thesocialjusticecentre.org/events/2020/5/15/organized -abandonment-cultures-of-crisis-and-resistance.

13. Niall McCarthy, "Nearly Three Times as Many Black Americans Are Dying from COVID-19 Compared with White People as Pandemic Death Toll Surpasses 150,000," *Forbes*, July 30, 2020.

14. As Salazar Vazquez notes in his piece, "From January to August 2020, ICE had approximated 450 deportation flights to fifteen different countries in Latin American and the Caribbean. Eleven of the fifteen countries reported that deportees arrived with COVID-19. These deportations contributed to the global spread of the virus, especially to a region that lacks the necessary resources to fight the pandemic. At one point, 20% of the total number of known COVID-19 cases in Guatemala were people deported from the United States. ICE's exportation of COVID-19 was so severe that the Honduran Ministry of Health required all deportees to be tested for COVID-19 upon arrival. Many of the deportees that tested negative later developed symptoms and tested positive."

15. In *Radical Skin, Moderate Masks: De-Radicalising the Muslim and Racism in Post-Racial Societies*, Yassir Morsi recounts his own efforts to determine whether or not a particular action is racist. Citing Salmaan Sayyid, he concludes that both enacting and detecting racism is a learned practice. Sayyid offers the example that immigrants who arrive in society that mark them as ethnically different may take years to understand that the way others react to them reflects an overarching racism (London: Rowman & Littlefield International, 2017: 125).

16. Louis Althusser, "Ideology and Ideological State Apparatuses (Notes Towards an Investigation)," in *Lenin and Philosophy and Other Essays*, trans. Ben Brewster (New York: Monthly Review Press, 1971), 142–47, 166–76.

17. Alyssa Paolicelli, "Mayor Seen in Video Turning Back on Chinatown Bakery Owner's Plea for Help," *Spectrum News NY1*, August 14, 2020.

18. Stacy Holman Jones, "Autoethnography: Making the Personal Political," in *Collecting and Interpreting Qualitative Materials*, ed. Norman K. Denzin, 3rd ed. (Thousand Oaks, CA: SAGE, 2008), 763.

19. Ibid., 764.

20. Layla D. Brown-Vincent, "Seeing It for Wearing It: Autoethnography as Black Feminist Methodology," *Communications on Stochastic Analysis* 18, no. 1 (September 19, 2019): 115.

21. Yassir Morsi, *Radical Skin, Moderate Masks*, 130.

22. Mahmood Mamdani, "Good Muslim, Bad Muslim: A Political Perspective on Culture and Terrorism," *American Anthropologist* 104, no. 3 (2002): 766–75.

23. In an effort toward representing my own situated positionality and autoethnographic sensibility, I am a non-Black Muslim woman of color, and my work focuses on anti-blackness as it intersects with the racialization of Muslims. Yassir Morsi, cited above, was a reader for my own dissertation defense. As with Morsi, I acknowledge that I can never assume the lived experience of anti-blackness, as I am not Black, and I am indebted to Black scholarship that has helped me understand my own processes of racialization and their enmeshment in white supremacy and racial capitalism. As Morsi notes in his autobiography, "I am wholeheartedly indebted to black scholarship. Without its long, illustrious, embodied and painful rejections of the terrors of racism (and without exaggeration), I would remain politically illiterate about who I am as a Muslim and person of colour." Morsi, *Radical Skin, Moderate Masks*, 9.

24. "The Inaction Timeline," Anti-Racist Coalition at Brooklyn College, https://antiracistcoalitionbc.wordpress.com/the-inaction-timeline/.

25. "CUNY Brooklyn College Student Population and Demographics," Univstats, 2021, https://www.univstats.com/colleges/cuny-brooklyn-college/student-population/.

26. https://antiracistcoalitionbc.wordpress.com/.

27. I have taken this formulation from Andrea Smith's "Indigeneity, Settler Colonialism, White Supremacy," in *Racial Formation in the Twenty-First Century* (Berkeley: University of California Press, 2012), 66–90. However I also wish to flag the controversy

surrounding Smith's problematic self-portrayal as Indigenous (Sarah Viren, "The Native Scholar Who Wasn't," *New York Times*, May 25, 2021).

28. "Are We Really 'All in This Together'? Challenging the Limits of Community," *CBC Radio*, September 9, 2020.

29. Mariame Kaba, "Yes, We Mean Literally Abolish the Police," *New York Times*, June 12, 2020.

30. Kathy Katella, "What Happens When You Still Have Long COVID Symptoms?," *Yale Medicine*, October 27, 2023.

31. From the poem "How to Explain White Supremacy to a White Supremacist," in Kyle "Guante" Tran Myhre, *A Love Song, A Death Rattle, A Battle Cry: Poems, Lyrics, and Essays by Kyle "Guante" Tran Myhre*, 2nd ed. (Minneapolis, MN: Button Poetry, 2017).

Chapter 11

1. Amy E. Cha and Robin A. Cohen, "Demographic Variation in Health Insurance Coverage: United States, 2020," Centers for Disease Control National Health Reports 169, February 11, 2022, https://www.cdc.gov/nchs/data/nhsr/nhsr169.pdf.

2. Rob Arnott, Vitali Kalesnik, Lillian Wu, "Collateral Damage from COVID," The Reason Foundation, October 2021, https://reason.org/wp-content/uploads/collateral-damage-of-COVID.pdf.

3. Annie Nova, "Millions of Americans Have Lost Health Insurance in this Pandemic-driven Recession," *CNBC*, August 28, 2020.

4. Arnott et al., "Collateral Damage from COVID."

Chapter 12

1. Gilbert C. Gee and Chandra L Ford, "Structural Racism and Health Inequities: Old Issues, New Directions," *Du Bois Review: Social Science Research on Race* 8, no. 1 (2011): 115–32.

2. "BIPOC Communities and COVID-19," Mental Health America, accessed July 15, 2023, https://mhanational.org/bipoc-communities-and-COVID-19.

3. Latoya Hill and Samantha Atiga, "COVID-19 Cases and Deaths by Race/Ethnicity: Current Data and Changes Over Time," KFF, August 22, 2022, https://www.kff.org/racial-equity-and-health-policy/issue-brief/COVID-19-cases-and-deaths-by-race-ethnicity-current-data-and-changes-over-time/; Irene Lew, "Race and the Economic Fallout from COVID-19 in New York City," Community Service Society, July 30, 2020, https://www.cssny.org/news/entry/race-and-the-economic-fallout-from-COVID-19-in-new-york-city.

4. Jordan M. Brooks, Cyrano Patton, Sharon Maroukel, Amy M. Perez, and Liya Levanda, "The Differential Impact of COVID-19 on Mental Health: Implications of Ethnicity, Sexual Orientation, and Disability Status in the United States," *Frontiers in Psychology* 13 (September 13, 2022).

5. https://taskeen.org/about/.

6. https://www.britishasiantrust.org/.

7. The 1947 Partition Archive, https://www.1947partitionarchive.org/.

8. Janet A. Liang. "Increasing Diversity Among Mental Health Care Providers Improves Trust and Reduces Cultural Stigma," AHA Institute for Diversity and Health Equity, July 26, 2022, https://ifdhe.aha.org/news/blog/2022-07-26-increasing-diversity -among-mental-health-care-providers-improves-trust-and.

Chapter 13

1. "NYCHA 2021 Fact Sheet," Nyc.gov, March 2021, https://www1.nyc.gov/assets /nycha/downloads/pdf/NYCHA-Fact-Sheet_2021.pdf.

2. Ibid.

3. "NYCHA Development Data Book 2020," Nyc.gov, Performance Tracking and Analytics Department, 2020, https://www.nyc.gov/assets/nycha/downloads/pdf/pdb 2020.pdf.

4. Susan J. Popkin and Mica O'Brien, "How Public Housing Authorities Are Support-ing Vulnerable Residents During COVID-19," Urban Institute, April 20, 2020, accessed July 20, 2023, https://www.urban.org/urban-wire/how-public-housing-authorities-are -supporting-vulnerable-residents-during-COVID-19; Tea Kvetenadze, "COVID Data Dearth at New York Public Housing Continues a Pattern of Neglect," Politico, Septem-ber 12, 2021, https://www.politico.com/news/2021/09/12/nyc-public-housing-residents -covid-511341.

5. Danielle Zielinski, "Chicago Public Housing: 'The Worst Place in the Country,'" *Daily Northwestern*, April 3, 2000.

6. Ibid.

7. Noah Goldberg, "At NYCHA's Most Dangerous Development, Tenants Wonder: Is the City Doing Enough?," *Brooklyn Eagle*, May 31, 2019.

8. Ibid.

9. Sara Dorn, "NYCHA Crime Surges as Harlem's Wagner Houses Become Gang Battleground," *New York Post*, September 15, 2019.

10. Greg B. Smith, "How Shootings Spiked at NYCHA Complexes Targeted in de Blasio Crime Prevention Campaign," *City*, February 1, 2021.

11. Pumla Kalipa, "South Bronx Gun Violence Spikes amid Pandemic," *Mott Haven Herald*, November 1, 2020.

12. Ibid.

13. "Staffer Delivering Food for Charity Shot on Upper West Side," *CBS News*, December 12, 2020.

14. A. Scott Henderson, "Tarred with the Exceptional Image: Public Housing and Popular Discourse, 1950–1990," *American Studies* 36, no. 1 (1995): 31–52.

15. Lisa Levenstein, *A Movement Without Marches: African American Women and the Politics of Poverty in Postwar Philadelphia* (Chapel Hill: University of North Carolina Press, 2009), 91.

16. Ibid., 91.

17. Rhonda Y. Williams, *The Politics of Public Housing: Black Women's Struggles against Urban Inequality* (New York: Oxford University Press, 2004), 222–23.

18. Ibid.

19. Ibid., 39

20. Edward G. Goetz, *New Deal Ruins: Race, Economic Justice, and Public Housing Policy* (Ithaca, NY: Cornell University Press, 2013), 39.

21. Ibid.

22. Helen Hershkoff and Stephen Loffredo, *Getting by: Economic Rights and Legal Protections for People with Low Income* (New York: Oxford University Press, 2020), 664.

23. Ibid.

24. Ibid.

25. "Policy Basics: Public Housing," Center on Budget and Policy Priorities, June 16, 2021, https://www.cbpp.org/research/public-housing.

26. Ibid.

27. Angelina Nelson, "NYCHA Residents Protest Pitfalls of Privatization," Epicenter, July 27, 2022, accessed November 16, 2022, https://epicenter-nyc.com/nycha-residents-protest-pitfalls-of-privatization/.

28. "Rental Assistance Demonstration-RAD," US Department of Housing and Urban Development (HUD), accessed June 28, 2023, https://www.hud.gov/RAD.

29. Nelson, "NYCHA Residents Protest Pitfalls of Privatization."

30. Ibid.

31. Harry DiPrinzio, "Hundreds of NYCHA Evictions Raise Questions About Process," *City Limits*, August 14, 2019.

32. Irene Lew, "The Pandemic Economy: COVID-19 Fallout Continues to Hit Low-Income New Yorkers the Hardest," Community Service Society of New York, November 19, 2020.

33. Ibid.

34. Dan Krauth, "7 on Your Side Investigates: New York City Eviction Notices Double, and Help Is Running Out," *ABC7 New York*, July 9, 2022.

35. David Brand, "NYC Eviction Rate Continues to Rise since Ban Was Lifted, as Homelessness Surges," *Gothamist*, January 18, 2023.

36. Eliza Shapiro, "Half of NYC Households Can't Afford to Live Here, Report Finds," *New York Times*, April 25, 2023.

Chapter 14

1. Malika Fair, "Why Is My Community Suffering More from COVID-19?" Association of American Medical Colleges, May 20, 2020, accessed July 20, 2023, www.aamc.org/news-insights/why-my-community-suffering-more-COVID-19; Clyde W. Yancy, "COVID-19 and African Americans," *Journal of the American Medical Association* 323, no. 19 (May 19, 2020).

2. K. Hinterland, M. Naidoo, L. King, V. Lewin, G. Myerson, B. Noumbissi, M. Woodward, L. H. Gould, R. C. Gwynn, O. Barbot, and M. T. Bassett, "Brooklyn

Community District 18: Flatlands and Canarsie," *Community Health Profiles 2018* 42(59):1–20.

3. Wikipedia. *The Narrows*. Wikipedia. https://en.wikipedia.org/wiki/The_Narrows.

4. Douglas Massey and Nancy Denton, *American Apartheid: Segregation and the Making of the Underclass* (Cambridge, MA: Harvard University Press, 1998).

5. Craig Wilder, *A Covenant with Color: Race and Social Power in Brooklyn, 1636–1990* (New York: Columbia University Press, 2000).

6. Ibid.

7. Ibid.

8. *Mapping Inequality: Redlining in New Deal America*, University of Richmond Digital Scholarship Lab, accessed October 9, 2021, dsl.richmond.edu/panorama/redlining /#loc=16/40.645/-73.961&city=brooklyn-ny&area=D15&adimage=3/57.327/-144.141; asylumprojects.org/index.php/Brooklyn_State_Hospital, Wilder, *A Covenant with Color.*

9. Massey, *American Apartheid.*

10. Themis Chronopoulos, "African Americans, Gentrification, and Neoliberal Urbanization: The Case of Fort Greene, Brooklyn," *Journal of African American Studies* 20 (2016), 294–322; Massey, *American Apartheid*; Wilder, *A Covenant with Color.*

11. Chronopoulos, "African Americans, Gentrification, and Neoliberal Urbanization."

12. "East Flatbush Neighborhood Profile," NYU Furman Center, retrieved November 11, 2022, https://furmancenter.org/neighborhoods/view/east-flatbush; "COVID-19 Data: Neighborhood Profiles," NYC Health, https://www.nyc.gov/site/doh/COVID /COVID-19-data-neighborhoods.page; "Flatlands/Canarsie Neighborhood Profile," NYU Furman Center, https://furmancenter.org/neighborhoods/view/flatlands-canarsie.

13. "Bay Ridge/Dyker Heights Neighborhood Profile," NYU Furman Center, retrieved November 12, 2022, https://furmancenter.org/neighborhoods/view/bay-ridge-dyker -heights; "COVID-19 Data: Neighborhood Profiles," NYC Health, https://www.nyc.gov /site/doh/COVID/COVID-19-data-neighborhoods.page

14. Derek Hyra, "The Back-to-the-City Movement: Neighborhood Redevelopment and Processes of Political and Cultural Displacement," *Urban Studies* 52, no 10 (2014); Chronopoulos, "African Americans, Gentrification, and Neoliberal Urbanization."

15. Karen Feldsher, "Pinpointing the Higher Cost of a Healthy Diet," *Harvard Gazette*, December 5, 2013.

16. Chronopoulos, "African Americans, Gentrification, and Neoliberal Urbanization"; "Bedford Stuyvesant Neighborhood Profile," NYU Furman Center, https://furman center.org/neighborhoods/view/bedford-stuyvesant; "Air Quality Data for NYC," Environment and Health Data Portal, retrieved November 12, 2022, https://a816 -dohbesp.nyc.gov/IndicatorPublic/beta/data-explore/air-quality/?id=2023#display= summary; Feldsher "Pinpointing the Cost"; "Restaurant Food Safety Data for NYC," Environment and Health Data Portal, https://a816-dohbesp.nyc.gov/IndicatorPublic /beta/data-explorer/restaurant-food-safety/?id=2065#display=summary,

17. "Asthma Data for NYC," Environment and Health Data Portal, https://a816 -dohbesp.nyc.gov/IndicatorPublic/beta/data-explorer/asthma/?id=2379#display=

summary; R. Bonita, R. Beaglehole, and T. Kjellstrom, "Basic Epidemiology," World Health Organization (2006); "Birth Outcomes Data for NYC," Environment and Health Data Portal, https://a816-dohbesp.nyc.gov/IndicatorPublic/beta/data-explorer/birth -outcomes/?id=5#display=summary; Wilder, *A Covenant with Color*.

18. "COVID-19 Data: Neighborhood Profiles," NYC Health, retrieved November 10, 2022, https://www.nyc.gov/site/doh/COVID/COVID-19-data-neighborhoods.page; "Fort Greene/Brooklyn Heights Neighborhood Profile," NYU Furman Center, https:// furmancenter.org/neighborhoods/view/fort-greene-brooklyn-heights; "Crown Heights/ Prospect Heights Neighborhood Profile," NYU Furman Center, https://furmancenter .org/neighborhoods/view/crown-heights-prospect-heights; "COVID-19 Data: Neigh-borhood Profiles," NYC Health, https://www.nyc.gov/site/doh/COVID/COVID-19-data -neighborhoods.page; "Bushwick Neighborhood Profile," NYU Furman Center, retrieved November 11, 2022, https://furmancenter.org/neighborhoods/view/bushwick; "Browns-ville Neighborhood Profile," NYU Furman Center, https://furmancenter.org/neighbor hoods/view/brownsville.

Chapter 15

1. John Paul, "'Flushing' Out Sociology: Using the Urinal Game and Other Bathroom Customs to Teach the Sociological Perspective," *Electronic Journal of Sociology* (2006).

2. C. Wright Mills, "The Promise," in *The Sociological Imagination* (Oxford: Oxford University Press, 1959), 3–24.

3. Octavia Butler, "A Few Rules for Predicting the Future," *Essence*, May 2000.

4. bell hooks, *All About Love: New Visions* (New York: William Morrow, 1999).

5. Mills, "The Promise," 13.

6. bell hooks, *Teaching to Transgress: Education as the Practice of Freedom* (New York: Routledge, 1994), 29.

7. hooks, *All About Love*.

8. Walidah Imarisha, Adrienne Maree Brown, and Sheree Renee Thomas, *Octavia's Brood: Science Fiction Stories from Social Justice Movements* (Chico, CA: AK Press, 2015).

9. Butler, "A Few Rules for Predicting the Future."

Chapter 16

1. Nick Niedzwiadek and Madina Touré, "SUNY, CUNY Halting In-Person Classes to Mitigate Coronavirus Threat," *Politico*, March 11, 2020.

2. Peter Whoriskey, Jeff Stein, and Nate Jones, "Thousands of OSHA Complaints Filed Alleging Companies Failed to Protect Workers from Coronavirus," *Washington Post*, April 16, 2020.

3. Jamie Ducharme, "World Health Organization Just Declared COVID-19 a 'Pan-demic.' Here's What That Means," *Time*, March 11, 2020.

4. Andrew Jacobs, Matt Ritchel, and Mike Baker, "'At War with No Ammo': Doc-tors Say Shortage of Protective Gear Is Dire During Coronavirus Pandemic," *New York Times*, March 19, 2020.

5. Nicole Acevedo, "Coronavirus: Puerto Rico needs medical supplies but faces restrictions." NBC News, March 21, 2020. See also Adriana M. Garriga López, "Compounded Disasters: Puerto Rico confronts COVID-19 under US Colonialism," *Social Anthropology* 28, no. 2 (2020): 269–70.

6. Clayton Skousen and Rose Hedges, "Olson Mask Pattern," UnityPoint Health, April 23, 2020, https://www.unitypoint.org/filesimages/COVID-19/UnityPointHealth-OlsonMask-Instructions.pdf.

7. Alan Mozes, "COVID-19 Ravages the Navajo Nation, but Its People Fight Back," *US News and World Report*, June 9, 2020.

8. Sahir Doshi et al., "The COVID-19 Response in Indian Country: A Federal Failure," Center for American Progress, June 18, 2020, https://www.americanprogress.org/article/covid-19-response-indian-country/.

9. Kim Gamel, "South Korea to Provide 10,000 Face Masks to Help Navajo Veterans Fight Coronavirus," *Stars and Stripes*, May 18, 2020.

10. "Coronavirus in Navajo Nation," CBS News, May 10, 2020, video, 27:05, https://www.cbsnews.com/video/coronavirus-in-navajo-nation/.

11. See Ericka Conant, "Puerto Rico's Hospitals Have Not Been Rebuilt More Than Three Years After Hurricane María," *Al Día*, May 28, 2021; Nicole Acevedo, "Coronavirus Worsens Food Insecurity in Puerto Rico–amid a Looming Loss of Federal Funds," NBC News, September 30, 2020.

Though I am referring to Puerto Ricans as US citizens in this section, I do not want to suggest that we are proud of that status. Rather, *if* the United States forced citizenship upon us while stripping us of a chance at becoming an independent nation, *then* it is their duty to ensure we live on—at least that is what is minimally expected. See also Yarimar Bonilla, "Postdisaster Futures: Hopeful Pessimism, Imperial Ruination, and La futura cuirm," *small axe*, 2020, 24 (2): 147–62.

12. Maureen O'Hare, "The World's Busiest Routes for February 2021," *CNN Travel*, February 10, 2021.

13. Mia Mingus, "You Are Not Entitled to Our Deaths: COVID, Abled Supremacy and Interdependence," *Leaving Evidence*, January 16, 2022, at https://leavingevidence.wordpress.com/2022/01/16/you-are-not-entitled-to-our-deaths-COVID-abled-supremacy-interdependence/.

Chapter 17

1. "Sunset Park Neighborhood Profile," NYU Furman Center, https://furmancenter.org/neighborhoods/view/sunset-park.

2. L. J. Dawson, "As Many Americans Get COVID-19 Vaccines and Financial Support, Undocumented Immigrants Keep Falling Through the Cracks," *Time*, March 8, 2021.

3. "New York included undocumented immigrants in pandemic aid, and 290,000 workers will benefit," Economic Policy Institute, May 19, 2021.

4. Tanvi Misra, "'We Have to Survive': Meet NYC Immigrant Women Fighting for Their Communities During the Pandemic," *The City*, October 3, 2021.

Chapter 18

1. For more on the protests in Trinidad, see Paul Hebert, "'70: Remembering a Revolution in Trinidad and Tobago," *Black Perspectives*, AAIHS, September 30, 2016, https://www.aaihs.org/70-remembering-a-revolution-in-trinidad-and-tobago/#.

2. Larry Buchanan, Quoctrung Bui, and Jugal K. Patel, "Black Lives Matter May Be the Largest Movement in US History," *New York Times*, July 3, 2020.

3. Madeline Drexler, "Deadly Parallels: Health Disparities in the COVID-19 Pandemic Mirror Those in the Lethal 1918 Flu," *Harvard Public Health*, Fall 2020, https://www.hsph.harvard.edu/magazine/magazine_article/deadly-parallels/.

4. Ibid.

5. Stuart Galishoff, "Germs Know No Color Line: Black Health and Public Policy in Atlanta, 1900–1918," *Journal of the History of Medicine and Allied Sciences* 40, no. 1 (1985), 26–27.

6. Ibid, 27.

7. Ibid.

8. Ibid, 29.

9. Vanessa Northington Gamble, "'There Wasn't a Lot of Comforts in Those Days': African Americans, Public Health, and the 1918 Influenza Epidemic," *Public Health Reports* 125, Association of Schools of Public Health, 2010, 114–22.

10. "Spanish Plague Raging in Chicago," *Chicago Defender*, October 9, 1918.

Chapter 19

1. Sharon Lerner, "'We Need Protein': Coronavirus Pandemic Deepens New York's Hunger Crisis." *The Intercept*, June 16, 2020.

2. Meal gap refers to the total annual food budget shortfall in an area divided by the weighted cost per meal in that area to account for differences in food costs and measure the extent of hunger in an area. "A New Survey of New Yorkers Exposes Pandemic Inequality: Unmasking the State of Hunger in NYC During a Pandemic," Food Bank NYC, June 2020, https://www.foodbanknyc.org/wp-content/uploads/Fighting-More-Than-COVID-19_Research-Report_Food-Bank-For-New-York-City_6.09.20_web.pdf.

3. Nimra Shahid and Marie Patino, "A New Survey of New Yorkers Exposes Pandemic Inequality," *Bloomberg*, February 24, 2021.

4. See Radical Living, https://radical-living.org/.

5. Shahid and Patino. "A New Survey of New Yorkers."

6. "Food Policy Organizations in Bedford/Stuyvesant," Hunter College New York City Food Policy Center, https://www.nycfoodpolicy.org/foodscape-bedford-stuyvesant/#references.

7. Jake Samieske, "Brooklyn's Unemployment Rate Decreases, but Is Still Higher Than NYC Average," *Brooklyn Magazine*, June 9, 2021.

8. Charles Platkin, "Testimony on the Status of Hunger in NYC and the Impact of COVID," NYC Food Policy Center, August 11, 2021, https://www.nycfoodpolicy.org/testimony-on-the-status-of-hunger-in-nyc-and-the-impact-of-COVID/.

Chapter 20

1. See: US Department of Labor, Office of Policy Planning, *The Negro Family: The Case for National Action*, Washington, DC: US Government Printing Office, 1965. This study challenged the prevailing logic that poverty resulted from the structure of society. The idea that was advanced was that due to slavery, the Black family represented a "tangle of pathologies." For a refutation of the Moynihan Report that argues that the Black family is the source of survival and achievement, see Andrew Billingsly, *Black Families in White America* (Englewood Cliffs, NJ: Prentice Hall, 1968).

2. Residential segregation is the sedimentation of US racism that is directly related to all other forms of inequality. W. E. B. Du Bois was perhaps the first to make this claim in his study of the predominantly Black Ninth Ward in Philadelphia in the late nineteenth century. His early identification of institutional racism would be eclipsed by the Chicago School of sociology that focused on the culture of ethnic groups and assimilation. See William Edward Burghardt Du Bois, *The Philadelphia Negro: A Social Study* (Philadelphia: University of Pennsylvania Press,1899). For a more recent critique of how the discipline of sociology purposely obscured the works of Du Bois, see Aldon Morris, *The Scholar Denied: WEB Du Bois and the Birth of Modern Sociology* (Oakland: University of California Press, 2015). Sociology would come around to Du Bois's findings almost a century later. See the seminal text: Susan Douglas and Denton Massey, *American Apartheid: Segregation and the Making of the Underclass* (Cambridge, MA: Harvard University Press, 1993).

3. Based on correspondence with Ebony during the drafting of this chapter, I was able to confirm that despite continued struggles she graduated two years later in the spring 2022 semester. She also gave birth to her child.

4. See Eduardo Bonilla-Silva, "Color-Blind Racism in Pandemic Times," *Sociology of Race and Ethnicity* 8, no. 3 (2022): 343–54. This is an extension of his earlier work: Eduardo Bonilla-Silva, *Racism Without Racists: Color-Blind Racism and the Persistence of Racial Inequality in the United States* (Lanham, MD: Rowman & Littlefield, 2006). For an informative article about dual pandemics see Ruqaiijah Yearby and Seema Mohapatra, "Law, Structural Racism, and the COVID-19 Pandemic," *Journal of Law and the Biosciences* 7, no. 1 (2020). Also intriguing is the relationship between the pandemic and the rise of white nationalism. See: Amanuel Elias, Jehonathan Ben, Fethi Mansouri, and Yin Paradies, "Racism and Nationalism During and Beyond the COVID-19 Pandemic," *Ethnic and Racial Studies* 44, no. 5 (2021): 783–93.

5. For a classic argument about how the social sciences do not accurately relate to Black communities see: Joyce Ladner, ed., *The Death of White Sociology: Essays on Race and Culture* (Baltimore: Black Classic Press, 1973). For a contemporary argument aimed specifically at methodologies see: Tukufu Zuberi and Eduardo Bonilla-Silva, eds., *White Logic, White Methods: Racism and Methodology* (Lanham, MD: Rowman & Littlefield, 2008).

6. See Patricia Hill Collins, "The Social Construction of Black Feminist Thought." *Signs: Journal of Women in Culture and Society* 14, no. 4 (1989): 745–73. This is a

specific example of how Black women are situated to know certain things based on their experiences.

7. See Hanes Walton, *Invisible Politics: Black Political Behavior* (Albany: State University of New York Press, 1985), which challenged the dominant political science view of behavioralism that froze Black communities as static, assuming institutional voting patterns and categories or individual decision process based on limited categories.

8. See Oscar Lewis, "The Culture of Poverty," *Scientific American* 215, no. 4 (1966): 19–25.

9. See Franklin D. Gilliam Jr., "The 'Welfare Queen' Experiment: How Viewers React to Images of African-American Mothers on Welfare." *Nieman Reports* 53, no. 2 (1999).

10. See Chapter 9 in Craig Steven Wilder, *A Covenant with Color: Race and Social Power in Brooklyn 1636–1990* (New York: Columbia University Press, 2000).

11. The following is the link that the students wrote to the Brooklyn College administration that prompted their visit to our class: https://drive.google.com/file/d/1K4sPt YT4-LHyPnbuhlr3V4uZxPOTu5_9/view?usp=drive_link.

12. The following link is the full letter from the students in the course: https://drive .google.com/file/d/1UzFmIGsi9Si3fUCBRwO0DfeUNmgsWuQW/view?usp=drive _link.

Chapter 21

1. This essay captures a moment in time of my experience of the pandemic. It was written between Spring 2020 and Fall 2022. In the Spring of 2023, when the lockdown period of the pandemic ended in Los Angeles and businesses reopened, I began working as a file clerk for a law firm. Also, my grandfather's health deteriorated, and we moved him into a nursing home.

2. "IHSS Program Data," California Department of Social Services, https://www .cdss.ca.gov/inforesources/ihss/program-data IHSS recipients are either Medi-Cal or Medicare recipients and some also receive Supplemental Security Income or State Supplementary Payments.

3. Ibid. In April 2021, Hispanic women made up 59.8% of IHSS recipients across California.

4. Ruben Vives, "San Fernando Valley's Latino Neighborhoods Staggered by LA County Virus Outbreak," *Los Angeles Times*, December 1, 2020.

5. Natalie Brouillette, et al., "It Changed Everything": The Safe Home Care Qualitative Study of the COVID-19 Pandemic's Impact on Home Care Aides, Clients, and Managers." *National Library of Medicine* 21 (2021), https://www.ncbi.nlm.nih.gov/pmc /articles/PMC8491760/. According to this article, the US Bureau of Labor Statistics predicts a more than 30% jump in the demand for home health aides and personal care aides over the next two decades.

6. "The US Population Is Aging," Urban Institute, https://www.urban.org/policy -centers/cross-center-initiatives/program-retirement-policy/projects/data-warehouse /what-future-holds/us-population-aging.

7. Sarah Thomason, et al., "California's Homecare Crisis: Raising Wages Is Key to the Solution." UC Berkeley Labor Center, November 2017, https://laborcenter.berkeley .edu/pdf/2017/Californias-Homecare-Crisis.pdf. See also, Naderah Pourat, "Home Care Quality and Safety: A Profile of Home Care Providers in California," UCLA Center for Health Policy Research, August 2013, https://healthpolicy.ucla.edu/publications /documents/pdf/homehealthreport-aug2013.pdf.

8. Deborah Schoch, "Study Shows 1 in 5 Americans Provide Unpaid Family Care," AARP, June 18, 2020.

9. Lai J. Kianbo et al., "Factors Associated with Mental Health Outcomes Among Health Care Workers Exposed to Coronavirus Disease 2019," *JAMA Network Open*, March 2, 2020, https://pubmed.ncbi.nlm.nih.gov/32202646/.

10. Eden Schulz, "Economic Impact of Family Caregiving: Families Caring for an Aging America," NCBI, November 8, 2016, https://www.ncbi.nlm.nih.gov/books /NBK396402/.

11. "Caregiving in the US 2020," AARP Public Policy Institute, https://www.aarp .org/ppi/info-2020/caregiving-in-the-united-states.html.

12. Ibid.

13. "Living Wage and Service Worker Retention Ordinances," Los Angeles World Airports, https://www.lawa.org/lawa-businesses/lawa-administrative-requirements/living -wage-and-service-worker-retention-ordinances

14. "The 2020-21 Budget: Department of Social Services," California Legislative Analyst's Office, February 24, 2020, https://lao.ca.gov/Publications/Report/4175 #IHSS.

15. Thomason et al., "California's Homecare Crisis."

16. Melissa Hunter et al., "COVID-19 Intensifies Home Care Workforce Challenges," ASPE, May 31, 2021.

17. Molly Kinder, "Essential but Undervalued: Millions of Health Care Workers Aren't Getting the Pay or Respect They Deserve in the COVID-19 Pandemic," Brookings, 28 May 2020.

18. Fay Gordon, "Special Report: Advocacy Starts at Home," Justice in Aging, February 2016, http://justiceinaging.org/wp-content/uploads/2016/02/FINALAdvocacy -Starts-at-Home_Strengthening-Supports-for-Low-Income-Adults-and-Family -Caregivers.pdf.

19. Linda Delp and Katie Quan, "Homecare Worker Organizing in California: An Analysis of a Successful Strategy," UC Berkeley Labor Center, https://laborcenter .berkeley.edu/wp-content/uploads/2020/09/DelpQuan.pdf.

Chapter 22

1. "California tops 10,000 coronavirus-related deaths," *Los Angeles Times*, August 7, 2020.

2. "Builders Nail Down an Exemption; Projects of All Sizes—Deemed Essential by State—Continue in LA Despite Pandemic," *Los Angeles Times*, April 26, 2020.

3. Samantha Brown, Raina D. Brooks, and Xiuwen Sue Dong. "Coronavirus and Health Disparities in Construction," Centers for Disease Control, 2020, https://stacks .cdc.gov/view/cdc/90044.

4. Ibid., 5. See also, "Are Construction Workers at Higher Risk for COVID-19 Complications?" Laborers' Health and Safety Fund of North America, August 2020, https://www.lhsfna.org/are-construction-workers-at-higher-risk-for-COVID-19 -complications/.

5. Joe Bousquin, "Construction Accounts for the Most COVID-19 Deaths of Any Industry in Colorado," Construction Dive, August 11, 2021. See also Will Huntsberry, "The First Year of COVID: Farm and Construction Workers Among Those Most Likely to Die," Voice of San Diego, December 16, 2021. The other industries with the highest proportionate rates of COVID-19 deaths of workers are transportation, warehousing, and agriculture—all industries with high percentages of Latinx workers.

6. US Bureau of Labor Statistics, "The Construction Industry: Characteristics of the Employed, 2003–20," April 2022.

7. New Americans in Los Angeles," New American Economy (December 16, 2021). Retrieved from: https://www.newamericaneconomy.org/wp-content/uploads/2017/02 /LABriefV8.pdf.

8. Ibid.

9. Daniel Cheriyan and Jae-Ho Choi, "A Review of Research on Particulate Matter Pollution in the Construction Industry," Journal of Cleaner Production 254 (May 2020).

10. Cora Roelofs et al., "A qualitative Investigation of Hispanic Construction Worker Perspectives on Factors Impacting Worksite Safety and Risk," Environmental Health 10, no. 1 (2011).

11. Ibid.

12. Leticia Saucedo and Maria Cristina Morales, "Masculinities Narratives and Latino Immigrants Workers: a Case Study of the Las Vegas Residential Construction Trades," Harvard Journal of Law & Gender 33, no. 2 (January 2010): 638.

13. Ibid, 639.

14. Ibid, 649.

15. "Home Building Continues amid Shortage; Construction Is Deemed Essential. but There Are More Gloves at Work Sites," Los Angeles Times, March 23, 2020.

16. Chukwuma Nnaji, Ziyu Jin, and Ali Karakhan, "Safety and Health Management Response to COVID-19 in the Construction Industry: A Perspective of Fieldworkers," Process Safety and Environmental Protection, 159, 477–88. See also, Remy F. Pasco, Spencer J. Fox, and S. Claiborne Johnston, "Estimated Association of Construction Work with Risks of COVID-19 Infection and Hospitalization in Texas," JAMA Network Open, October 29, 2020.

17. Ibid.

18. Shelly Stiles, David Golightly, and Brenda Ryan, "Impact of COVID-19 on Health and Safety in the Construction Sector," Human Factors and Ergonomics in Manufacturing & Service Industries 31, no. 4 (January 12, 2021): 425–37.

Chapter 23

1. Institute for Women's Policy Research, "Student Parents In COVID-19 Pandemic: Heightened Need and the Imperative for Strengthened Support," April 14, 2020, https:// iwpr.org/wp-content/uploads/2020/07/COVID19-Student-Parents-Fact-Sheet.pdf.

2. Ibid.

3. Paul Ong, "COVID-19 and the Digital Divide in Virtual Learning," UCLA Center for Neighborhood Knowledge (Fall 2020), https://escholarship.org/uc/item/07g5r002.

4. California Department of Education, "Muir K–8, 2020–2021 School Accountability Report Card," https://sarconline.org/public/print/19647256015531/20202021?CFID= 43958015.

5. A 2016 study found that, "among people with incomes under the national median, 41 percent of foreign-born Hispanics with children said that they only ever accessed the internet via mobile device. . . . Similarly, 44 percent of immigrants who are Hispanic did not use a computer at all . . . compared to 19 percent of US-born Hispanics, a rate similar to other ethnic groups." Alexis Cherewka, "The Digital Divide Hits US Immigrant Households Disproportionately During the COVID-19 Pandemic," Migrationpolicy.org, September 3, 2020, https://www.migrationpolicy.org/article/digital-divide-hits-us-immigrant-households-during-COVID-19.

6. Sidney Johnson, "Thousands of California Students Still Without Laptops and Wi-Fi for Distance Learning," *EdSource*, April 7, 2020, https://edsource.org/2020/thousands-of-california-students-still-without-laptops-and-wi-fi-for-distance-learning/628395.

7. Kyle Stokes, "Coronavirus Exposed a 'Digital Divide' in LA Schools. See Where That Gap Is Widest," *LAist*, April 6, 2021, https://laist.com/news/coronavirus-digital-divide-map-los-angeles-distance-learning. See also, Brooke Auxier and Monica Anderson, "As Schools Close Due to the Coronavirus, Some US Students Face a Digital 'Homework Gap,'" Pew Research Center, 27 July 2020.

8. Ibid.

9. Ibid.

10. Ibid.

11. Paulette Cha and Niu Gao, "The Digital Divide Has Narrowed but Still Affects California's Children," Public Policy Institute of California, August 10, 2012, https:// www.ppic.org/blog/the-digital-divide-has-narrowed-but-still-affects-californias-children/.

12. Jie Park et al., "Educating Children and Navigating Digital Literacy in COVID-19: Latina Mothers and Mother-Child Pedagogies," *International Journal of Multicultural Education* 23, no. 3 (2021): 79–93.

13. Madeleine Bair and Ashley McBride, "With Online Schooling, Latino Immigrant Parents Fear Their Kids Are Being Left Behind," *Oaklandside*, October 26, 2020, https://oaklandside.org/2020/10/09/with-online-schooling-latino-immigrant-parents-fear-their-kids-are-being-left-behind/. See also, Nicole Acevedo, "Latino Parents Face

Back-to-School Uncertainty as COVID-19 Hits Their Families Hard," NBCNews.com, August 3, 2020, https://www.nbcnews.com/news/latino/latino-parents-face-back-school -uncertainty-COVID-19-hits-their-n1235439

14. Park et al., Ibid.

15. Ibid.

16. This was a widespread problem among undocumented immigrants, who because of unemployment and income loss during the pandemic, were unable to provide their children with internet access, or for whom "lock-downs in high-density households may result in sharing devices, interference from family members, and reduced Internet speeds. Lockdowns may also prevent individuals from accessing community support networks for developing digital literacy." Zach Bastick and Marie Mallet-Garcia, "Double Lockdown: The Effects of Digital Exclusion on Undocumented Immigrants During the COVID-19 Pandemic," *New Media & Society* 24, no. 2 (2022): 365–83. See also Juan Carlos Gomez and Vanessa Meraz, "Immigrant Families During the Pandemic: On the Frontlines but Left Behind," CLASP: Center for Law and Social Policy, February 11, 2012, https://www.clasp.org/publications/report/brief/immigrant-fami lies-pandemic-frontlines.

17. Sumit Chandra, et al., "Closing the K–12 Digital Divide in the Age of Distance Learning," Common Sense Media and Boston Consulting Group (2020). See also, Enrico Gandolfi, Richard E Ferdig, and Annette Kratcoski. "A New Educational Normal an Intersectionality-Led Exploration of Education, Learning Technologies, and Diversity During COVID-19," *Technology in Society* 66, no. 6 (2021).

18. Organisation for Economic Co-operation and Development, "What Is the Impact of the COVID-19 Pandemic on Immigrants and Their Children?," October 19, 2020, https://www.oecd.org/coronavirus/policy-responses/what-is-the-impact-of-the-COVID -19-pandemic-on-immigrants-and-their-children-e7cbb7de/. See also, Pauline Barto-lone, "Hundreds of Sacramento Kids Stopped Schooling Due to COVID-19," CapRadio, June 2, 2020, https://www.capradio.org/articles/2020/06/02/hundreds-of-sacramento -kids-stopped-schooling-due-to-COVID-19/.

Chapter 24

1. County of Los Angeles Department of Public Health, "Safer at Home Order for Control of COVID-19," April 10, 2020, downloaded at https://COVID19.lacounty.gov /wp-content/uploads/HOO_Safer-at-Home-Order-for-Control-of-COVID_04102020 .pdf.

2. Elisa Facio, "Spirit Journey: 'Home' as a Site for Healing and Transformation," in *Fleshing the Spirit: Spirituality and Activism in Chicana, Latina, and Indigenous Women's Lives*, edited by Elisa Facio and Irene Lara (Tucson: University of Arizona Press, 2014); 60. For a discussion of "safe space" for undocumented LGBTQ people, see Jesus Cisneros and Christian Bracho, "Undocuqueer Stress: How Safe Are 'Safe' Spaces, and for Whom?," *Journal of Homosexuality* 67, no. 11 (2020): 1491–511.

3. Gilbert Gonzalez et al., "Mental Health Needs Among Lesbian, Gay, Bisexual, and Transgender College Students During the COVID-19 Pandemic," *Journal of Adolescent Health* 67, no. 5 (2020): 647. For research on mental health concerns of LGBT+ Latinos prior to the COVID-19 pandemic, see Nicole N. Gray et al., "Community Connectedness, Challenges, and Resilience Among Gay Latino Immigrants," *American Journal of Community Psychology* 55, nos. 1–2 (2015): 202–14.

4. Kerith J. Conron, Kathryn O'Neill, and Brad Sears, "COVID-19 and Students in Higher Education," UCLA School of Law Williams Institute, May 2021, https://williams institute.law.ucla.edu/publications/COVID-19-college-students/.

5. Laura E. Enriquez et al., "COVID on Campus: Assessing the Impact of the Pandemic on Undocumented College Students," *AERA Open* 7 (July 20, 2021).

6. Ibid.

7. Gloria Anzaldua, *Borderlands/La Frontera: The New Mestiza* (San Francisco: Aunt Lute Books, 1987).

8. Editor's note: The Spanish word "joto" is a pejorative term for gay men. These terms have been reclaimed by queer and trans Chicanx and Latinx activists and scholars in the United States to signify cultural pride and political empowerment and resistance. By using this term in their essay, the author is situating their work within the emergent academic field of Jotería Studies. See Michael Hames-García, "Jotería Studies, or the Political Is Personal," and Anita Tijerina Revilla and José Manuel Santillana, "Joteria Identity and Consciousness," both in *Aztlán: A Journal of Chicano Studies* 39, no. 1 (2014).

Chapter 25

1. Students' names were changed to protect their privacy, and they consented to my sharing this information in this essay.

2. In 2021–22, 72% of Cal State LA students were Latinx, the vast majority of Mexican or Central American heritage. This was the highest percentage of any four-year university in California and was surpassed only by a few colleges in Texas and Puerto Rico. "Hispanic-Serving Institutions (HSIs) 2021–22," Hispanic Association of Colleges and Universities (HACU), https://www.hacu.net/images/hacu/OPAI/2023_HSILists.pdf.

3. June Jordan, "Report from the Bahamas" (1982) from *Some of Us Did Not Die: New and Selected Essays* (New York: Civitas Books, 2003).

4. Lidia Marte, *Cimarron Pedagogies: Notes on Auto-ethnography as a Tool for Critical Education* (New York: Peter Lang, 2020), 2.

5. Cindy Cruz, "LGBTQ Youth Talk Back: A Meditation on Resistance and Witnessing," *QSE: The International Journal of Qualitative Studies in Education* 25, no. 5 (2014), 547–58.

6. Linda Tuhiwai Smith, *Decolonizing Methodologies: Research and Indigenous People* (New York: Zed Books, 2001).

7. Maria Lugones, *Pilgrimages/Peregrinajes: Theorizing Coalition Against Multiple Oppressions* (Lanham, MD: Rowman & Littlefield, 2003), 7.

8. Julie Livingston, "To Heal the Body, Heal the Body Politic," in *The Long Year: A 2020 Reader*, ed. Thomas J. Sugrue and Caitlin Zaloom (New York: Public Books, 2022), 231.

9. For academic studies of Latinx communities and COVID-19, see: Natalia Molina, "The Enduring Disposability of Latino Workers," in Sugrue and Zaloom, *The Long Year: A 2020 Reader*; Edward D. Vargas and Gabriel R. Sanchez, "COVID-19 Is Having a Devastating Impact on the Economic Well-Being of Latino Families," *Journal of Economic, Race, and Policy* 3 (2020): 262–69; and Maria Elena Martinez and Jesse Nodora, "The Dual Pandemic of COVID-19 and Systemic Inequalities in US Latino Communities," *Cancer* 127, no. 10 (2021).

10. "Los Angeles County Case Summary," Los Angeles County Department of Public Health, August 22, 2022, http://publichealth.lacounty.gov/media/Coronavirus /locations.htm#case-summary.

11. Edwin Flores, "LA County Sees a Latino Mortality Rate Increase of 48 Percent During Pandemic," NBC News, April 15, 2022, https://www.nbcnews.com/news/latino /l-county-sees-latino-mortality-rate-increase-48-percent- pandemic-rcna24622.

12. Alicia Victoria Lozano, "'The gaps widen': In hard-hit LA, Latinos Bear the Brunt of COVID's Surge," NBC News January 17, 2021, https://www.nbcnews.com/news/us -news/gaps-widen-hard-hit-l-latinos-bear-brunt-COVID-s-n1254342.

13. Luis Noe-Bustamante, Jens Manuel Krogstad and Mark Hugo Lopez, "For US Latinos, COVID-19 Has Taken a Personal and Financial Toll," Pew Research Center, July 15, 2021, https://www.pewresearch.org/race-ethnicity/2021/07/15/for-u-s-latinos -COVID-19-has-taken-a-personal-and-financial-toll/.

14. In Sugrue and Zaloom's *The Long Year*, an edited collection of forty-nine essays about the pandemic by some of the world's most notable scholars, not one focused squarely on the problem of segregation. Similarly, among dozens of articles published in the *Los Angeles Times* and *New York Times* about COVID and racial disparities in LA County, only one op-ed substantively discussed residential segregation as an historical and present cause of inequitable health resources in non-white areas of LA.

15. Juan Onésimo Sandoval, Hans P. Johnson, and Sonya M. Tafoya, "Who's Your Neighbor? Residential Segregation and Diversity in California," Public Policy Institute of California, August 2002, https://www.ppic.org/wp-content/uploads/CC_802JSCC.pdf.

16. Jill Cowan and Matthew Block, "In Los Angeles, the Virus Is Pummeling Those Who Can Least Afford to Get Ill," *New York Times*, Jan 29, 2021.

17. Nadia Kim, *Refusing Death: Immigrant Women and the Fight for Environmental Justice in LA* (Stanford, CA: Stanford University Press 2021), 12.

18. Erica Yee et al., "How Big Is California's Historic Budget, Visualized," Cal Matters, June 12, 2022, https://calmatters.org/politics/2022/06/california-budget-surplus -explained/.

19. John Fensterwald, "California Is 36th in nation in *Education Week*'s latest rankings in per-student spending," *Ed Source*, June 14, 2021, https://edsource.org/updates/cali fornia-is-36th-in-nation-in-education-weeks-latest-rankings-in-per-student-spending.

20. M. Jaqui Alexander, "Not Just (Any) Body Can Be a Citizen: The Politics of Law, Sexuality and Postcoloniality in Trinidad and Tobago and the Bahamas," *Feminist Review*, no. 48 (Autumn 1994): 12.

21. Leah E. Daigle, Katelyn P. Hancock, and Travis Chafin, "Covid-19 and Its Link to Victimization Among College Students," *American Journal of Criminal Justice* 46.5 (2021), 683–703.

22. In *Pilgrimages/Peregrinajes*, Lugones describes a "faithful witness," as one who "witnesses against the grain of power, on the side of resistance," 7.

Conclusion

1. We are using the first-person plural "we" in the conclusion rather than "they" (the student authors) to convey the immediacy of the conversation, the urgency for change, as well as the ways this project and the ideas generated are a sum greater than its parts. We are using "we" to connote the collective call for reflection about what needs to change, but have tried to mark the places where the "we" includes experiences students had that we did not and to be cognizant of our different subject position in the pandemic.

CONTRIBUTORS

Alan Aja is professor and chair in the Department of Puerto Rican and Latino Studies and codirects the Mellon Transfer Student Research Program with Jeanne Theoharis and Joseph Entin at Brooklyn College. His scholarly work in economic stratification is a means for activism and action for universal, collective goods. His recent book with Michelle Holder, *Afro-Latinos in the US Economy*, statistically explores the material realities of the US Afro-Latinx population. Alan plays basketball regularly, enjoys coaching youth soccer, nerds out about green public transportation across global cities, and dreams of tuition-free public university systems.

Anthony Almojera is an EMS Lieutenant and vice president of Local 3621, the New York Fire Department EMS Officers' Union. Anthony is a twenty-year veteran working in the NYC EMS system, and the author of *Riding the Lightning; A Year in the Life of a New York City Paramedic*, his engrossing memoir published by Harper Collins in 2022.

Adia Atherley was born and raised in Brooklyn, New York, and history and human interactions have always been particularly interesting to her. She is a graduate student at Brooklyn College with a focus in history.

Dominick Braswell is an activist from Brooklyn, New York. Graduating from Brooklyn College with a degree in Africana Studies, he is a doctoral student in Afro-American Studies at the University of Massachusetts–Amherst. Dominick's research focuses on the history of public housing and how race has influenced attacks on the program.

Zayd Brewer stubbornly wields a pen in a world of ever-sharpening swords. Writing comes more naturally to him than most things. He also raps under the alias Spaceman and finds music to be a suitable means of expression.

Wendy Casillas is a queer, gender-nonconforming, Mexican-American individual and a graduate of California State University, Los Angeles. They double-majored in women's gender and sexuality studies and anthropology. Their life mission is to spread awareness on issues focused on improving the lives of BIPOC and LGBTQ+ people.

Maria Cerezo graduated from Cal-State LA with the class of 2023 and is starting a job helping the East LA community. She enjoys a good true-crime documentary as well as spending time with her family. Maria hopes to one day obtain her masters in the field of mental health.

Tania Darbouze's life experience has been centered around her background and upbringing as a Haitian American who grew up in Flatbush, Brooklyn. This nurturing has brought her to being a graduate of Brooklyn College and an active mutual aid organizer, now working in fire rescue operations in California.

Marsha Decatus earned a BS in biology and MPH from the State University of New York at Albany (SUNY), where she discovered how systemic inequality determined health outcomes among society's most marginalized populations. Moved by this challenge, she returned to her hometown, Brooklyn, New York, to begin her work toward health equity—completing a fellowship with the New York State Department of Health (NYSDOH), AIDS Institute. Marsha turned to Brooklyn College to complete her health prerequisite courses while continuing to work toward health parity in her favorite borough.

Joseph Entin has been teaching English and American studies at Brooklyn College since 2003. He is the author or coeditor of five other books, including *Living Labor: Fiction, Film, and Precarious Work* (2023). He is also a long-time member of the *Radical Teacher* editorial board and a co-founder of the Brooklyn College Listening Project.

Donna-Lee Granville is a sociologist who studies race, immigration, and culture and teaches courses like Sociology of Hip Hop, Urban Caribbean Diaspora, and Consumer Society and Culture. In her spare time, Dr. Granville can be found sharing insights and laughs on Twitter and TikTok or organizing TEDxFlatbush events.

Kayla Gutierrez is a half-Chinese and half-Dominican woman, who grew up in Chinatown in a predominantly Chinese cultural household. She graduated from Brooklyn College in 2021 with a major in English and a minor in history and has an interest in archival/preservation work.

Manuel (Manny) Ibarra is a nonbinary, first-generation, Chicanx born in Michoacan, Mexico. They are a DACA student attending Graduate School at Cal State Los Angeles in the Chicanx and Latinx Studies Department with the end goal of obtaining a PhD. Their area of focus is the intersectional aspect of Queer and POC communities, in particular the pedagogies of the home for queer undocumented individuals.

Billie-Rae Johnson graduated in 2020 with a bachelor's degree in urban sustainability from Brooklyn College. She is passionate about people and the environment and actively advocates for the just treatment of both. Some of her interests include creative writing, anime, minimalism, and music—and her dream is to see the world.

Lawrence Johnson is a sociology professor who specializes in race and politics. He maintains that the trajectory of sociology hinges not solely upon its subject matter, but also upon the innovative approaches employed in its teaching and application. His current research explores how high school football has been utilized by coaches on the South Side of Chicago as a form of resistance, while simultaneously being used by elite stakeholders to perpetuate urban restructuring and displacement.

Elizabeth Leon Lopez is a CSULA alumna who graduated with a bachelor's in liberal studies. She is currently working on her multiple-subject teaching credential and hopes to someday earn a master's in early child development.

Alejandra Marchevsky is a professor of women's, gender, and sexuality studies at Cal State LA. She is a Latina immigrant scholar-activist whose work critically interrogates gendered racism and state violence, focusing on Latinx migrants in the United States. Her publications explore gendered migration from Latin America and Latinx labor in the United States, the carceral logics of the US welfare and immigration systems, and African American and Chicana coalition building in the welfare rights movement.

Genesis Orea is a Brooklyn native who graduated from Brooklyn college in 2020 with a BA in political science and a minor in Puerto Rican and Latino studies. Her work has been focused on immigrant communities, postsecondary education, and her dog, Luna. Genesis is currently enrolled as a law student at CUNY School of Law and hopes to graduate with her JD in 2026.

Yamilka Portorreal graduated from Brooklyn College in 2021 with a major in urban sustainability and a minor in environmental science. They're originally from the Dominican Republic, and in their spare time they like to experiment in visual arts using the mediums of photography and drawing. They now work in agricultural research regarding climate change.

Rhea Rahman is an assistant professor of anthropology at Brooklyn College. Her research and teaching centers on global logics of racialization and forefronts the question: how is human difference used for justifying systems of inequality and oppression, and how might we instead engage difference with an eye toward liberation? Rahman is currently working on a manuscript that frames international Muslim volunteerism, humanitarianism, and development through intersecting logics of global white supremacy, anti-Muslim racism, and anti-Blackness.

Samantha Saint Jour is a Haitian-American Canarsie, Brooklyn, native. She spends most of her time writing personally and academically and exploring different career paths. Most of all, Samantha loves her community, staying close to home in her role as Brooklyn College's Black Student Union graduate advisor.

Anthony Salazar Vazquez is a born-and-raised New Yorker from Mexican immigrant parents. He received his BA in Puerto Rican and Latino studies from CUNY Brooklyn College. Currently, he pursues ways to continue his education in Latin America, Caribbean, and Latino studies.

Jeanne Theoharis is distinguished professor of political science at Brooklyn College and the author or coauthor of eleven books on the Black freedom struggle and the contemporary politics of race in the United States. Her widely acclaimed biography *The Rebellious Life of Mrs. Rosa Parks* won a 2014 NAACP Image Award and has been adapted into a documentary of the same name, directed by Johanna Hamilton and Yoruba Richen and executive produced by Soledad O'Brien for NBC-Peacock, where she served as a consulting producer.

Raúl Vaquero is a Mexican-American ENL educator fueled by his own multilingual journey. His passion lies in exploring the ideological intersections of race and language within American education, particularly in the context of second-language acquisition and bilingual education.

Daniel J. Vázquez Sanabria is a PhD candidate in the Department of Mexican American and Latina/o Studies at the University of Texas at Austin. His work examines how cultural productions of disability in Puerto Rico manifest and are shaped by language, intracommunity conflicts, cultural politics, and colonial discourses. He is often floating through the transmarikona soundscapes of Villano Antillano's musical repertoire.

Khadhazha Welch's upbringing in the Trinidad and Tobago countryside cultivated a strong bond with nature and a commitment to community impact. Guided by her grandparents' teachings, she is dedicated to environmental stewardship and policy change.

Areeba Zanub is a Pakistani-American writer and artist who graduated from CUNY Brooklyn College with a BA in English. Outside of academia, she enjoys poetry, painting, and photography. Infused with a vibrant blend of Pakistan and New York City, she aspires to bridge connections between the two and inspire South-Asian Americans through her work.

INDEX

ACKNOWLEDGMENTS

We still can't believe we have gotten to bring this book into the world.

At each stage, this project has exceeded our wildest imagination: that we got the initial pandemic research grant from the Social Science Research Council (SSRC); that eighteen students in that first harrowing summer were so courageous and driven to make sure that there would be a record of what was happening in Brooklyn; that *Black Perspectives* wanted to publish not one, not two, but eight of that first group's pieces; that Brooklyn College was able to fund the second cohort of twelve students and the Mellon Foundation, excited about the project and research by students, funded a third cohort; that Alma Gottlieb, faculty editor of the "Contemporary Ethnography" series at the University of Pennsylvania Press, and then press editor Jenny Tan reached out because they thought it could be a book; that Alejandra Marchevsky, inspired by what we were doing, asked her own students in Los Angeles to write autoethnographies, which they did with such astounding results; that twenty students on two coasts were willing to do the courageous and painstaking work of revising their pieces for the public. Wow. Simply wow. We feel so fortunate to get to do this.

This project has changed us immeasurably in several ways, particularly in how deeply we see and feel the impacts of the pandemic around us. Working on this project with these students has meant years of combining anger, sorrow, determination, and hope at how the devastating and rolling consequences of the pandemic and the preexisting social conditions that contributed to its devastation are minimized and individualized with the urgency of how this society needs to reckon with that and to change. Over decades of teaching at Brooklyn College we have learned that our students have the perspectives, imagination, and insights our society desperately needs and we, along with many of our colleagues, have come to see our primary job as supporting our students to become their most powerful selves. It has been one of the great honors of our lives to get to do this book with our students and colleagues.

There are so many people to thank:

Our first thanks go to Dominick Braswell, whose insights and ideas helped form the basis for the application we submitted to SSRC, and who provided the logistical and community-building assistance for each of the three cohorts of student writers. This project simply would not exist without him. Dominick and Kayla Gutierrez provided key research and bibliographic assistance as we turned this into a book. Jasmaine Brathwaite played an invaluable role in creating community in the cohorts of student writers. The three of them helped lay the groundwork for the success of this project.

We owe a huge debt of gratitude to Alondra Nelson, former head of the SSRC, who helped initiate the rapid-response grants for research on inequality and the pandemic. She understood that these students could produce needed research and then came to our first conference and listened and engaged deeply with our students and their ideas and writing.

Much of our work with students over the last several years, and on this project in particular, has been made possible by generous grants from the Mellon Foundation for the Mellon Transfer Student Research Program, which we codirect with Alan Aja. We are immensely grateful to the people at the Mellon Foundation we have worked with—Earl Lewis, Eugene Tobin, Dianne Harris, Armando Bengochea, and Susan Dady—who have grasped the significance of funding humanities research initiatives for students at CUNY. Support from Mellon has been transformative for us, for our students, and for Brooklyn College.

This book only exists because Jenny Tan and Alma Gottlieb had the idea in the first place. We have published many books and know scores of colleagues who have. We have *never* heard of a book that centered the perspectives and framings of working-class public college students of color. Alma's and Jenny's visions that this could be a book—that this *needed* to be a book—have made this volume possible. There are not sufficient words to mark our deep gratitude for their imagination and leadership. We also want to thank copyeditors Jon Dertien and Gary Hamel, as well as Lily Palladino from the press, who helped sharpen the prose and shepherd the book into production.

An enormous note of thanks goes to Keisha Blain and Tyler Parry, who saw the rich perspectives and urgent need to publish this student work in the fall of 2020 in *Black Perspectives*, the blog of the African American Intellectual

Society. Without this *Black Perspective* series, there would be no book and probably no additional student cohorts after the first one in 2020.

We are grateful to Brooklyn College and the Brooklyn College Foundation, including Brooklyn College President Michelle Anderson and Vice President for Institutional Advancement Todd Galitz, for funding to support a cohort of student writers in January 2021.

We are grateful to all the students who took part in the three cohorts of this project. As we note in the introduction, they all produced amazing work, but most of that work does not appear in this book. To write about the often-painful details of one's life and the life of one's family, during a time of pandemic struggle and strain, is a daunting task. And then to revise and revise again and again, and to make that writing public, is doubly difficult. This book is suffused with the energy, intelligence, courage, fortitude, and insights of all the students we worked with whether or not their writing appears in these pages. We thank them for sharing their stories with us and their peers in the summers of 2020 and 2021, and in January 2021. Our introduction brims with what we learned from and experienced with all these students. Beyond them, we are grateful to all the students who have participated in the Mellon Transfer Student Research Program over the years. Their smarts, intellectual bravery, and commitment to research has taught us so much about the world and about the questions that need to be asked and the research that needs to be pursued to transform society. Alan Aja, our fellow MTSRP codirector and co-facilitator of the third cohort, has played an invaluable role in this book, our spirits, and the mentoring that produced the work in this book. Alan's ideas about student power and his commitment to public education have infused our work on this book and our days at the college.

We have been fortunate to have Richard Greenwald, Ken Gould, Rosamond King, and Phil Napoli as deans, and Jennifer Matisi as their executive coordinator. They have been some of our biggest cheerleaders and supporters and we are grateful for the way they have backed us, our work, and our students.

We are deeply indebted to the faculty who have provided the responses for the five sections in this book: Alan Aja, Rhea Rahman, Donna Granville, Lawrence Johnson, and Alejandra Marchevsky. Over many conversations and revisions, they have helped us imagine the book that this has become. We owe particular gratitude to Alejandra Marchevsky, who brought her Cal State L.A. students into this project. Her work with them, her dedication to them and her thinking about this project and its stakes and implications have shaped and sharpened our own understandings. And her commitment to truth-telling and tremendous heart have buoyed our own vision and spirit. We are also grateful to the three anonymous peer reviewers who heartily endorsed the project and offered insights that helped us revise. We also want to express our gratitude to colleagues and friends who read versions and talked with us about this project, including Irene Sosa, Gaston Alonso, Phil Napoli, Naomi Schiller, Jocelyn Wills, Jessica Siegel, María Pérez y González, Carolina Bank Muñoz, James Davis, Ellen Tremper, Alexandra Juhasz, Naomi Braine, Mobina Hashmi, and Prudence Cumberbatch. Beyond them, we are grateful to all our CUNY comrades who are supporting our students and fighting to secure the full public funding our students deserve.

Writing is always a collective effort—this project especially! For us, friends and family have provided the essential support that has kept us going during the challenging political and social times during which this project came into being. They have listened over and over throughout the many years of this project—as we struggled with what we were seeing in the first autoethnographies, processing what it meant to make space for this kind of truth telling, and kept going through many difficult spells. Profound thanks to Sophie Bell, Miriam and Rachel Entin-Bell, Audrey Entin, Lena Entin, David Entin, Dorothy Riehm, Claudia and Walter Gwardyak, Cathleen Bell, Rick Kahn, Steve O'Neill, Alejandra Marchevsky, Arnold Franklin, Liz Theoharis, George Theoharis, Say Burgin, Aviva Stahl, Toni Rodriguez, Stephanie Melnick, Carl Hart, Gayatri Patnaik, Karen Miller, Erik Wallenberg, Melissa Madzel, Jason Elias, and Robyn Spencer.

This book is a testament to the power of collaboration—and the strength and insight that are gained by working collectively. We are grateful to be doing this together. Holding space for all this project entailed would have been psychically impossible alone.

Our greatest thanks go to the students, whose brave and beautiful framings lay bare how much our country has failed during the pandemic. Doing some of the hardest writing we have ever had the privilege to be part of, they demonstrate how the inequalities that the pandemic brought into relief were not happenstance but by design. At the same time, they reveal the values around which a new world could be built, the love that makes surviving through these searing inequities possible, and the kinds of policies that would reflect the just and compassionate society we all deserve. We hope this book helps to carry that vision forward.